If it's better health, good sex and long life you seek—let *100 Days* be your guide

Life is your single greatest possession. Without it, money, big houses and fancy cars mean little. To this end, humankind has always sought ways to achieve better health and increased longevity. And perhaps none were more successful than the Taoists of ancient China—who often lived to be well over 100 years old.

Now, Eric Steven Yudelove's latest book captures these ancient secrets in a 100-day program of Chi Kung, Taoist health, sexual yoga, self-massage rejuvenation, and longevity practices. These practices are not religious, but they are often quite different from what we are used to. And this is the first time that much of this knowledge is available to Western readers.

Presented in a 14-week format, *100 Days to Better Health, Good Sex & Long Life* introduces you to the power of Chi Kung, the Six Healing Sounds, Baduanjin, Self-Massage, Sexual Kung Fu, the Inner Smile, Opening the Golden Flower, and much more. You'll be doing authentic Taoist practices in the very first week!

If you seek harmony and balance in your otherwise hectic world, take 15 minutes out of your day and let *100 Days to Better Health, Good Sex & Long Life* be your guide.

about the author

Eric Steven Yudelove (New York) has studied Taoist practices since 1970. In 1981 he was one of the first American students to study with Mantak Chia, an authentic Tao Master. In 1983 Mr. Yudelove became one of the original certified instructors in the Healing Tao, and is currently a senior instructor. He is also a practicing trial lawyer and the author of *The Tao & the Tree of Life*.

to write to the author

If you wish to contact the author or would like more information about this book, please write to the author in care of Llewellyn Worldwide and we will forward your request. Both the author and publisher appreciate hearing from you and learning of your enjoyment of this book and how it has helped you. Llewellyn Worldwide cannot guarantee that every letter written to the author can be answered, but all will be forwarded. Please write to:

Eric Steven Yudelove
c/o Llewellyn Worldwide
P.O. Box 64383, Dept. K833-8
St. Paul, MN 55164-0383, U.S.A.

Please enclose a self-addressed stamped envelope for reply, or $1.00 to cover costs. If outside U.S.A., enclose international postal reply coupon.

100 DAYS TO BETTER HEALTH, GOOD SEX & LONG LIFE

A GUIDE TO TAOIST YOGA & CHI KUNG

Eric Steven Yudelove

1997
Llewellyn Publications
St. Paul, Minnesota 55164-0383 U.S.A.

FIRST EDITION
First Printing, 1997

Cover design: Tom Grewe
Interior design and editing: Michael Maupin
Illustrations: Carrie Westfall

Library of Congress Cataloging-in-Publication Data
Yudelove, Eric Steven.
   100 days to better health, good sex & long life: a guide to taoist yoga / Eric Steven Yudelove.--1st ed.
     p. cm.
   Includes bibliographical references and index.
   ISBN 1-56718-833-8 (trade paper)
   1. Hygiene, Taoist. 2. Chi kung. 3. Health. 4. Longevity
 5. Hygiene, Sexual. I. Title.
RA776.5.Y83 1997
613--dc20   97–33493
                                CIP

Publisher's Note:
Llewellyn Worldwide does not participate in, endorse, or have any authority or responsibility concerning private business transactions between our authors and the public.

   All mail addressed to the author is forwarded but the publisher cannot, unless specifically instructed by the author, give out an address or phone number.

The practices, techniques, and meditations described in this book should *not* be used as an alternative to professional medical treatment. This book does not attempt to give any medical diagnosis, treatment, prescription, or suggestion for medication in relation to any human disease, pain, injury, deformity, or physical condition.

   The author and publisher of this book are not responsible in any manner whatsoever for any injury which may occur through following the instructions contained herein. It is recommended that before beginning the practice you consult with your physician to determine whether you are medically, physically and mentally fit to undertake this course of practice.

Llewellyn Publications
A Division of Llewellyn Worldwide, Ltd.
P.O. Box 64383, Dept. K833-8
St. Paul, MN 55164-0383, U.S.A.

acknowledgments

The author wishes to thank Mantak Chia for helping to make this book possible. Much of the material in *100 Days to Better Health, Good Sex & Long Life* is derived from my fifteen years of study with Master Chia as a student, an instructor, and a senior instructor for The Healing Tao.

I thank Healing Tao Books and Juan Li for allowing me to redraw many of the illustrations found in this book.

I wish to acknowledge Aurora Press for publishing Mantak Chia's first two books: *Awaken Healing Energy through the Tao* and *Taoist Secrets of Love: Cultivating Male Sexual Energy*. Much of the oral teachings that I learned directly from Master Chia were subsequently written down in both of them.

I wish to thank Master Yun Xiang Tseng for his assistance in providing me with an accurate picture of Chi Kung as it is currently practiced in China.

I wish to thank all of the authors listed in the bibliography. Each one of them furthered my knowledge of the Tao.

In *100 Days to Better Health, Good Sex & Long Life* I have done my best to present an accurate description of Chi Kung and the practices of the Taoists. The manner and form of its construction is uniquely my own and I ultimately bear responsibility for its success or failure.

contents

WEEK SIX

Breath

Body

Mind

WEEK SEVEN

Breath

Body

Mind

WEEK EIGHT

Breath

Body

Mind

WEEK NINE

Breath

Body

Mind

WEEK TEN

Breath

Body

Mind

WEEK ELEVEN

Breath

Body

Mind

WEEK TWELVE

Breath

Body

Mind

WEEK THIRTEEN

Breath

Body

Mind

WEEK FOURTEEN

exercises

introduction

WHAT IS YOUR GREATEST POSSESSION? Do you believe that it's your house, or your car or your jewelry? Is it your collection of fine stamps or rare coins or your investment portfolio? Possessing any or all of these things can improve the quality of your life. But could any of them truly be called your greatest possession?

Maybe you believe that your greatest possession is not actually a thing at all. Maybe it's your sense of humor or your charm. Maybe it's your personality or your golf swing. Maybe it's the well-tuned ear of the music lover or the well-trained nose and tongue of the wine expert or gourmet. Maybe it's some talent you have that makes you unique. These are our possessions too. And although any of them can help to define who we are or who we think we are, can any of them truly be called our greatest possession?

Maybe you believe that your greatest possession is your job, or your drive to succeed. Maybe it's your thirst for knowledge or your ability to communicate. Maybe it's your ability to read. Maybe it's your television set.

Each person has different possessions that help to define who and what they are. Your greatest possession may be something you don't even have yet but are sure you will someday obtain. It may be your religious belief. For some it's their family, for others, the respect of their peers.

Your greatest possession can mean different things to different people. It would certainly be difficult to get people to agree on any one thing or quality that all people would consider to be their greatest possession.

Our concept of our greatest possession is based on many variables. How we were brought up, who our parents were, and what values we were given are certainly important. Whether we were raised in a big city or small town or on a farm or in the mountains isolated from society would all play a major role in determining our concept of what is our greatest possession.

The perfect baseball swing of a boy raised in the United States would be of little value to a boy raised in India.

When we seek a definition of what is our greatest possession, we must arrive at something that has a more universal acceptance.

We may possess great riches but, if we become seriously ill we realize that good health is more valuable than dollars. And although being rich may help us to get better medical treatment, it is our health itself which is ultimately a greater possession than money or things.

We may possess many talents but, if we are seriously depressed or mentally ill, we cannot appreciate them. If you lose your mental well-being or know someone who has, it is easy to see that all the riches in the world are meaningless or worthless if your mind is not intact.

So health and mental well-being are certainly universally recognized as great possessions. But, even underlying these two is something more basic. It is something we take with us everywhere we go. It is something we can lose or sacrifice, it is something we can waste or give away. It is also something that we can make great use of and take great care of. Ultimately, it is our greatest possession. It is our life.

Your life is your single greatest possession. If you lose it, all your other possessions or talents are worthless to you. If you are dead, then the concept of possessing something becomes meaningless. Your memory may live on in your family and friends. The things you have accumulated during your life will pass on to your heirs, but without life, you possess nothing.

Life is thus our greatest possession and it is also our greatest gift. We received life from our parents and we possess the ability to create life in our children. This is a great and wonderful gift—the gift of life. And life itself is ultimately a great mystery. Our science still cannot tell us where life comes from and where life goes when it is over. The source of life really defies logical explanation. Call it God, or nature, or Tao. Ultimately, we are faced with the unanswerable question of where God came from or how nature could conceive itself. All we can say with certainty is that life exists here on planet Earth and that humans appear to be the highest form of life on our planet.

Life itself has two basic functions. From the point of view of nature, the function of life is the preservation of the species. In the greater scheme of things, the continuation of the human race through the process of reproduction is more important than the preservation of individual life. However, from the point of view of us individuals, self-preservation is our greatest possession.

We carry our life around with us in the vehicle we call our body. In order to preserve our body, we must breathe and receive nourishment.

In order to be truly human, we must also nurture another aspect of life which is called consciousness. Humanity has the gift of awareness of the world and universe around us. This is what separates humans from all other forms of life. We can think creatively. We can question our existence. We create languages and writing and mathematics. We are aware of our emotions and have created laws defining good and evil, what is acceptable and unacceptable in our society.

As we reach the end of the twentieth century, science and medicine have succeeded in extending life expectancy and eradicating many dangerous diseases. We also benefit from the exchange of ideas about health and longevity from all over the world.

Western medicine is still relatively young. Its emphasis has been more on curing illness than prevention. As we head into the twenty-first century, we will find that the healing arts and sciences will expand in scope to encompass new and old ideas from all over the world.

To that end, I dedicate this book. In it, I will write about the healing, longevity, rejuvenation and sexual techniques originally developed by the Taoists in ancient China. Many of the Taoist practices have just begun to be revealed in the West. Until the late 1970s, there were virtually no Tao Masters in the West. The Taoists lived in China, often in remote locations. They had no reason to ever leave China until the Taoist practices were suppressed during the Communist Revolution and even more violently during the Cultural Revolution in the late 1960s.

Those who were able fled mainland China for other parts of the Orient. From Taiwan, Hong Kong, Thailand, etc., the teachings were spread first to the Chinese communities and then to the population at large. Eventually, the teachings arrived in America in the form of Tao Masters such as Mantak Chia and Hua Ching Ni.

Taoist practices were renewed in China in the 1970s as the government came to realize that so much of the Taoist cultural inheritance had virtually been annihilated in China. Taoist exercises called Chi Kung are now practiced all over China. Tai Chi Chuan is practiced in parks every morning by millions of Chinese. Medical doctors in China learn Taoist techniques. Scientists and universities study the Life Force Energy called Chi in hopes of better understanding the mysteries of life. A new generation of Chinese Chi Kung masters have appeared, some of whom have been allowed to travel to the West and teach.

I was fortunate to begin studying with Master Mantak Chia in 1981 soon after his arrival in the West from Thailand. I have continued my studies until the present time, not only with Master Chia but with numerous practitioners, masters and students from all over the world. In this book, I will do my best to cut through the technical aspects of the practice. Of course, it will be necessary to explain the basic Taoist concepts of health and longevity which have a definite Oriental mindset. However, the techniques and practices are universal in appeal and require no prior knowledge of Chinese philosophy, science or medicine.

The approach will be practical and I will try to keep things as simple as possible. Simplicity is a Taoist virtue. I am obviously not Chinese. I cannot speak or read Chinese. I am a Western man who has studied and practiced Taoist techniques for more than twenty years. My aim here is not to explain the workings of the Oriental mind to the West, but rather to bring many highly beneficial health, rejuvenation, longevity, and sexual techniques out into the open so that people from all walks of life can learn them and live longer, healthier and more enjoyable lives.

There are many excellent books on the market that explain who the Taoists were, give their history and legends and explain their beliefs. If you are interested, by all means go out and read them. In the present book, I will keep the background to a minimum. One word of caution though: there were many different Taoist schools of thought. Many of the teachings are open to different interpretations and points of view. If you read too much, all at once, you're apt to get confused with all the differing viewpoints. Remember to keep things simple.

The Taoist practices are not religious. They comprise physical and mental exercises that are often quite different from those we are used to in the West. To the Taoists, long life and good health were primary concerns. Many of the exercises and practices are simple and easy to perform. This book is a practical approach to the healing, sexual, rejuvenation, and longevity techniques of the Taoists. The Taoists sought to extend life as long as possible. Possessions and material wealth were not necessarily shunned by the Taoists but life was definitely their greatest possession.

The Taoist techniques of health, rejuvenation, longevity and sexuality are great possessions. Once you learn them, you can take them with you wherever you go. They require no special equipment or apparatus. They are fully portable but weigh nothing. In their ability to transform and rejuvenate your life, maintain your health, increase your longevity and improve your sex life, they could well become your most precious possession.

道

part one

道

Background to the Practice

The Goal of Good Health and Long Life

THROUGHOUT HISTORY, HUMANKIND HAS SOUGHT ways to achieve better health and increase longevity. The Taoists of China achieved great success in both of these endeavors.

Until recently, the health and longevity practices of the Taoists were unknown in the West. There were many reasons for this. For one, the Taoists tended to live in remote parts of China. Many of their teachings were handed down as secrets and were not available to even the general Chinese population. The teachings that were written down were often done so in a cryptic manner so they were basically unintelligible even to the Chinese. Few of these texts were ever translated into English and those that were required great effort and study to gain even a glimmer of the ideas and processes that the Taoists practiced.

Luckily, much of the mystery has now been cast aside as true Tao Masters have begun teaching in the West. Also, the opening of China and the free flow of information has greatly increased our knowledge of these wonderful techniques and practices.

Still, aside from the philosophy of the Taoists, little of their practices has trickled down to the general population, and this is unfortunate. Part of the problem is in the perception that only martial artists or health food fanatics could benefit from the study and practice of the Taoist techniques. And although martial artists will greatly benefit from the practice, and a healthy diet can enhance success, in truth everyone could benefit from some aspect of the teachings.

Another problem has been the difficulty in presenting these Oriental concepts to the West. Chinese concepts of the body, health and mind are often quite alien to Western thinking. Much of what has been written in the West has been either highly technical or overwhelming in approach.

The health, sexual, rejuvenation and longevity practices of the Taoists grew out of their quest for immortality. They believed that through the process of Taoist Internal Alchemy, it was possible to develop an immortal spirit body that could actually leave the physical body and exist independently. Taoist history is filled with stories of such immortals. The term "immortal" also came to be applied to practitioners of the Tao who achieved extreme old age. Often, the terms were interrelated. The process of internal alchemy required many years to perfect so that it was necessary to live a very long life before the achievement of immortality was possible. Physical exercises, breathing exercises and techniques of controlling the mind were developed to help the would-be immortal to maintain his strength and physical well-being long enough to achieve the production of the immortal spirit body. As they developed, it was recognized that aside from the quest for immortality, the exercises, practices and techniques actually promoted good health, rejuvenation and long life aside from any spiritual quest. In this book, we will explore many of these practices as they relate to health, rejuvenation, longevity and sexuality.

Extreme old age among Taoists was common. There are legends of ancient Taoists who lived many hundreds of years, sometimes thousands of years. These stories, of course, cannot be confirmed. But, modern history records the story of Li Ching-Yuen who was born in the seventeenth year of the Ching Dynasty or A.D. 1678 in Szechuan Province in China. In 1749 at age 71, he joined the army. He spent most of his life in the mountains and was married fourteen times. In 1927, General Yang Sen met with and photographed Li Ching-Yuen and became his disciple. The following year, Li Ching-Yuen died at the age of 250 years. After his death, General Yang investigated the facts of Li Ching-Yuen's life and found them to be truthful. Li Ching-Yuen had three basic rules to achieve long life: 1) Avoid all types of emotional extremes. These drain the body of energy and disrupt the harmonious functioning of the body's organs. This is especially true of older people. 2) Don't hurry through your life. Take your time, don't rush. 3) Practice physical and breathing exercises (Chi Kung) daily.

I cannot guarantee that following Li Ching-Yuen's rules will lead to extreme old age. His disciple General Yang died young at the age of 98.

To begin the actual practice of Taoist techniques, we must adopt our own Three-Pronged Approach. This involves regulating l) the breath, 2) the body, and 3) the mind. The Taoist practices are integrated. We don't do only physical exercises. We don't do only breathing exercises. We don't do only mental exercises and meditation. We do all three and we combine all three. This is necessary to build a firm foundation for ourselves. In this book, we will learn how to build that firm foundation in the practices of the Tao.

What Is the Tao?

There is something magical and wonderful about the word *Tao*. Its modern spelling is Dao, but I prefer the old way: Tao.

The Tao translates into English as *the Way*. To explain the Tao to a Westerner is very difficult. The Way includes everything you've ever thought about. The Way includes everything you've never thought about. Nature follows the Way. The Way includes all concepts of God that humans have created or worshipped. The Way controls the course of the universe.

But, what does any of this mean? Ultimately, the Way or the Tao is something that cannot be defined. Tao is a word that is really a symbol for something that underlies all of reality. But we are told that the Tao that can be written about is not the real Tao. You see we have a problem here with language. There is no word or set of words in English that can define the Way because it is indefinable. The Tao includes everything. It includes all words, all thoughts and all actions.

The Tao is something you experience by learning to exist in harmony with it. The Way includes the force of the Earth and the force of Heaven. Practicing the Tao teaches us to harmonize ourselves with the Way. This is why we must learn to regulate or harmonize our bodies, our breath and our mind. We must bring all the different facets of ourselves together as a unified being, an integral being.

The Tao symbolizes the totality of all things. It is a cosmic thought. Everything is connected as you expand your awareness to understand and wonder at the enormity of the Way. The Way is awareness. The Way encompasses good and evil and is bigger than both of them.

When you practice the Way, you feel connected. You feel grounded to the Earth. A Taoist learns to deal with his or her own energy and the energy of the Earth. One who walks on the Way learns to control his or her own energy. This lies at the heart of the practice of the Tao.

Probably the best term to call these practices would be *Taoist Yoga*. In China, it is generally referred to as *Chi Kung*. Actually, Chi Kung is just a part of Taoist

Yoga. Taoist Yoga is taught by a Tao Master. The true Tao Masters are literally extinct in China. In their place we have Chi Kung Masters who have lost the sexual secrets and internal alchemy but have made a science of the study of Chi. Chi Kung is a vital part of Taoist Yoga and in this book we will not be dealing with Internal Alchemy. So, you can call these practices Chi Kung or Taoist Yoga, whichever you prefer. In English we call them Energy Exercises.

Chi Kung

Kung refers to any training or study that requires a real effort over a sufficient period of time. Chi Kung means any training or study dealing with Chi that requires a lot of effort spread out over a long period of time.

Chi is another one of those magical words that find no true English equivalent. But, really, for this book, Chi is the Key. There are many ways to spell Chi or Chee. The modern translation is Qi. In Japan it is called Ki. Chi, Chee, Qi, or Ki, it's all the same energy, just different spellings. I like Chi best myself, but you are welcome to use any spelling of any of the Chinese words in this book as you prefer. Many of these words have multiple transliterations into English.

Everyone in China understands the basic concept of Chi. But, in the West, the concept of Chi seems to stump even some of our greatest minds. I'll try my best to describe Chi. Literally, Chi means air. Chi Kung originally referred to practitioners of breathing exercises. Regulation of the breath is one of the three prongs of the practice of the Tao, the other two being regulation of the body and regulation of the mind.

Chi has a host of other meanings with different shadings and changing qualities. From breath, the meaning expands to the breath of life or the life force. It is the energy of life. So, Chi Kung also means the study and practice of the Life Force Energy. For our purposes, Chi is both our breath and our life force. The two are intimately related. Just think, if you stop breathing for only a few minutes, your life force will leave you.

In this book, we will also refer to Chi as Energy. I want to take some of the mystery out of the practice of the Way by removing as much of the Oriental trappings and symbolism as possible. The ideas here are really universal. The basic concept is to learn to control your Life Force Energy.

We all recognize that all living creatures possess the life force. In the West, I know of no specific study that deals with the training of the life force. Our sports and athletics train the body and the breath and doctors now recognize that some form of exercise will help you to live longer. The Taoists developed these exercises into a science and an art form.

The Taoists looked at life from a different perspective than did Westerners. Taoist scientists explored the Life Force Energy (Chi). They found that they could use their minds to learn to control the Chi. They found they could use breath to control the Chi. They also learned that Chi could be moved in the body by different types of physical exercises. The Taoist combined breath and mind and found new ways to control the Life Force Energy. Moving exercises using both the breath to control and the mind to direct the Chi were created. As their Chi was regulated and harmonized, the Taoists learned to move the Life Force Energy with the mind alone. In this book, we will explore all these ways to control and direct the Life Force Energy.

Energy Circulation

Just as our body has a circulatory system for the transportation of blood, it also has a Chi or Energy circulatory system.

Chi moves throughout the body in what are known as channels or meridians. These channels were mapped out long ago by the Chinese medical community and are an integral part of traditional and modern Chinese medicine. They are most popularly known as acupuncture meridians in the West. But acupuncture is actually a means of altering the flow of Chi through the channels using thin needles.

Our bodies have thirty-two main channels through which Chi flows. In the two primary channels, Chi flows up the spine and over the head in the Governor Channel (Du Mai) and down the front of the body in the Functional Channel (Ren Mai). Most of the other thirty channels begin in the fingertips or toes and flow into and through the body.

What we are talking about here is simply the flow of energy through the body. Everyone has this Life Force Energy. Although the principles of this energy flow were discovered in the East, there is nothing inherently Chinese about the energy itself. Western science recognizes the meridian system of Chi flow even if it is not well understood. It is not mysticism. It is science. As we move into the twenty-first century, this system will become better known and eventually will be integrated into Western medicine. Modern Western medicine is actually only a few hundred years old. The knowledge of the flow of Chi through the channels has been known in China for thousands of years.

Jing: The Essence

Our major source of Chi comes from the various forms of liquids, fluids and hormones produced in our body. This includes the blood, the lymph system, all hormones secreted by glands in our body and male and female sexual fluids and hormones including the sperm and the egg. Taken as a unit they are all referred to as *Jing*, or Ching. In English this translates to "Essence." This is a difficult concept for many Westerners. To use a graphic example, if we were turned into wet sponges, what you could squeeze out of us would be our Essence, our Jing. It is the Essence of our life.

Jing is not the same as Chi. Essence is not the same as Energy. The body converts Essence into Energy. Essence, or Jing, is something that is often tangible and can be seen or felt. Energy, Chi, cannot as yet be seen or measured.

Jing also refers to the essential nature of all things. Everything has Jing, be it living, dead, organic or inorganic. Essence is used here in terms of what gives something its unique quality and character. For instance, a rock has rock Jing, a dog has dog Jing, the sun has sun Jing, the moon has moon Jing, your heart has heart Jing, etc. Jing can take on an infinite number of forms.

We absorb the Essence of the food we eat and convert it to Chi that supplies the energy needs of our body. Food and breath are our two main outside sources of Jing.

As we age, the primary interior source of Jing in our bodies comes from the sexual organs. In men it is found in the semen and related male sexual hormones and in women it is in the ova and the female related sexual hormones. The sexual Jing is converted into a powerful form of Chi inside of the body. As we reach puberty and young adulthood, the sexual Essence converted into sexual Energy becomes the body's primary driving force. By middle age and later, when our sexual potency begins to wane, our energy levels begin to decrease substantially.

The Taoists realized that for men, the loss of semen used up vast amounts of Jing. This happens each time a man ejaculates. The Taoists developed many techniques to conserve sexual Jing and to convert more of this Essence into Chi. Some of these techniques are quite simple and will be discussed later in the practice section of this book.

Women lose Jing mainly during menstruation. Between a man and a woman having equally active sex lives, the man will lose more Jing. Taoists believe that this is a major reason, on average, women live longer than men. They have more Essence available for conversion into Energy. We will also explore techniques for women to conserve and convert their Essence. Hereon we will refer to sexual Jing as Jing Chi.

Original Energy

Everybody receives their Original Essence from the union of their mother's ova with their father's sperm cell. The Taoists called this Original Essence—Yuan Jing. The amount and quality of Original Jing is different in each person. We each have a finite amount of Original Essence. It will sustain us through our lives. Taoists consider it to be our most important treasure. To sustain and preserve our life, we must conserve our Original Jing. In order to stay alive and grow, Original Jing must be converted into Original Chi. In other words, we receive the Original Essence of who and what we are, our Original Nature, from our parents' egg and sperm. Original Essence is converted into our Original Life Force Energy. This Original Chi (Yuan Chi) provides the spark of life. It maintains the embryo as it grows in its mother's womb and keeps it healthy.

The amount of our Original Jing determines the amount of our Original Chi. The amount of our Original Essence determines the amount of our Original Life Force. As used here, the two terms Original Essence and Original Chi are practically interchangeable and in effect determine the quality and length of our lives. When we are young, it is our Original Jing and Chi that sustain us. Original Jing is constantly being converted into Energy. However we can use up and waste our Original Essence. This is why the Taoists trained to strengthen the Jing and conserve it. When it is all used up, we die.

Original Chi also had another meaning. Inside of its mother's womb, the growing fetus never takes a breath of air, yet the Original Chi flows cleanly and unimpeded through all its Energy Channels. The fetus receives nourishment to sustain the Energy flow through the umbilical cord which is attached to it at the navel.

Once the child is born and the umbilical cord is cut, it begins to breathe. Air now becomes a major source of Chi for the infant along with the liquid nourishment it receives from its mother's milk or baby formula. Eventually, the infant will begin eating solid foods and this too will become a major source of Chi.

The Taoists differentiated between the Original Energy and all other forms of Chi (remember Chi and Energy mean the same thing). Original Chi will sustain the fetus. It will be strong in the infant. As the infant grows into a child the Original Energy will be, normally, still strong. But as the child grows older and becomes a teenager and young adult, the strength of the Original Chi will slowly begin to wane. It will not flow quite as smoothly. As the adult ages, the strength of this Original Chi will continue to gradually weaken until finally, in old age, there is none left.

We can see that Original Energy carries us and sustains us throughout our lives, from the moment of conception until the moment of our death. The Taoists had many names for this Original Energy: Embryonic Chi, Prenatal Chi, Pre-Heavenly Chi and Primordial Breath are just some of them.

All other forms of Chi are referred to as Post-Natal Chi or Post-Heavenly Chi. These come from our Jing (especially Sexual Essence), the air we breathe and the food we eat.

Many of the Chi Kung practices are designed to restore the free flow of Energy throughout the body's Energy Channels. The basic concept is to restore that same flow of Original Chi that existed in you when you were a fetus in your mother's womb and did not even have to breathe to keep the Chi flowing smoothly. This is what Original Chi means to most practitioners of Chi Kung.

The Third Treasure

The Tao is the source of everything. Chi and Jing, Energy and Essence, are two great treasures from the Tao. There is one other treasure that along with Chi and Jing are known as the Three Treasures of Taoist Yoga. This Third Treasure is *Shen*.

Shen is another word that is difficult to translate into English. It includes all the activities of our mind including consciousness, thinking, dreaming, personality and ego. On another level it means Spirit. The Taoists believed that this was the part of us that could gain immortality. Many of the highest practices of Tao Masters involved working with the Spirit. Just as Jing is converted into Chi, Chi can be converted into Shen.

For our purposes, Shen will be equated with the mind and our mental faculties. All exercises involving thinking, concentrating, visualizing or meditating are exercises involving Shen.

The Three Treasures are our source of health, rejuvenation and longevity. They provide the means for our Three-Pronged Approach to the Taoist techniques which involve regulation of the breath, body and mind. We can now see that breath relates to Chi, the body relates to Jing and the mind relates to Shen. So now, when we mention Energy, Essence or Mind, please understand that we are referring to the Three Treasures given to followers of the Way. And when we do breathing exercises, physical and sexual exercises or mental exercises, we are, in fact, exercising our Three Treasures. Practicing Chi Kung involves the control, conservation, and increase of our Energy, Essence and Mind.

Yin and Yang

Here are two words that absolutely baffle us Westerners. Their most common meaning is woman and man. I've heard them used as slang for the sex act, such as "he's good in the yin-yang." The words are well known in the West, but what do they mean?

The key to understanding Yin and Yang is to realize that there is always an underlying third member that is the silent partner. This third member represents balance and harmony. The Taoists call it Tai Chi. Yang balances Yin. Yin balances Yang.

Tai Chi also means unity. The Yin and the Yang come together and give up their individuality to form a unit. The simplest example of this is a man and woman joining together to form a family. The family is the underlying concept of the Chinese way of life. Two people come together to form something new and bigger than either one of them individually. This, too, is Tai Chi.

In Chi Kung we seek balance and harmony in our breathing, in our body and in our mind to maintain ourselves and our greatest possession, our lives. So when we talk about Yin and Yang we're really talking about getting ourselves well balanced.

Everybody understands that in order for something to be in balance, there must be something to balance. For instance, on a see saw, the high end balances the low end. The high end is considered Yang and the low end Yin. In the Tao, Heaven, which is high, balances the Earth, which is low. This is Tai Chi.

In our body we must balance the Yang Chi received from our father's sperm cell at conception with the Yin Chi we received from our mother's egg. We acquired equal parts male and female at conception and the genetic markers in our chromosomes determined if we would grow up male or female. The point to remember is that our Original Chi was created from equal doses of Yin and Yang.

In Chi Kung, Yin and Yang manifests not so much as male and female, but as active and receptive. One part gives, the other receives. In our body's blood circulatory system, blood leaves the heart in arteries (active–Yang) and returns to the heart in veins (receptive–Yin). The arteries and the veins balance each other to form the circulatory system. This is Tai Chi.

We're closing in on grasping the concept of Yin and Yang. Any two thoughts, ideas, concepts, actions, activities, etc., that are opposed to, or balance each other, form a Yin-Yang relationship. Thus we have hard (Yang) and soft (Yin), day (Yang) and night (Yin), Heaven (Yang) and Earth (Yin), positive (Yang) and negative (Yin), hot (Yang) and cold (Yin) and white (Yang) and black (Yin) as a few examples.

Yin and Yang seek balance. In our bodies this balance is often lost. Our Original Chi kept our Yin and Yang Chi in balance. But as the strength of the Original Chi weakens, it loses the ability to keep us in perfect balance. We are more affected by the food we eat and the quality of the air we breathe, by the thoughts we think, the games we play and the medicines we take. When the body loses its original perfect balance, this affects the flow of Chi through the Energy Meridians in our bodies. Channels become blocked or constricted. That perfect flow of Energy, which used to run through all the Channels in our body, stops flowing quite so smoothly. You might feel it in your leg, or your back or in your neck. As you age you experience the loss of Chi flow as pain, numbness or stiffness. Chi Kung was created to help restore the free flow of Chi in the Energy Channels and to maintain the balance of Yin and Yang in the body.

For our purposes, think of Yin and Yang as the two poles of a battery. One pole is negative and the other positive. Together they work to keep the body and its component parts in balance. If one pole goes out of balance, it must be adjusted by an infusion of more energy from the opposite pole. For instance, if the body gets too hot (Yang) it must be cooled down with cold Yin energy. We can refer to these two types of Chi as Fire Energy and Water Energy or Yang Chi and Yin Chi. Our upper body, above the navel, where our major organs reside, is considered Yang and our lower body, below the navel, is Yin.

It's important to keep this simple. Chinese doctors spend years learning all the subtleties of balancing Yin and Yang in our bodies. It can get quite complex and is not necessary to know to begin the practice of Taoist Yoga.

The Gods of the Body

Many of us in the West expend a great deal of time and energy trying to get to know ourselves. We explore our psyche and often pay good money to do it.

To the Taoists, getting to know yourself means something entirely different. What we think of as ourselves is only something that we have created. Our ego is self-created. The Taoist understands that he or she was not born with an ego and when they die it will disappear, nowhere to be found. The Taoist learns to ignore the ego and little by little its hold is broken. This allows our Original Nature (Original Essence), our true self, to shine through and regain control of our lives.

Our Original Mind (Yuan Shen) came from the Original Essence (Yuan Jing) converted into Original Life Force Energy (Yuan Chi) at conception. Our Original Mind possessed no ego. When we were born, we had no thoughts. Thoughts came later, after we learned words.

The process of Chi Kung involves revitalizing and restoring our Original Chi. It is a process of rejuvenation. Part of the procedure involves restoring the Original Mind. This mind had no ego, no thoughts, no self-awareness. So gradually we attempt to regain that state of mind that we all once had, where the ego is not the dominating force in our brain. The ego is something we created as we grew up. It is not the real mind. The real mind is silent. The Taoists called this silence Nothing. To silence the mind is one of the higher goals of Chi Kung.

To really grow in the Way, it is necessary to look at life from a different perspective. This doesn't mean that you must give up what you believe in. No. Just be open-minded. Sometimes it is good to look at the world through the silent eyes of a child. It looks completely different.

To a Taoist's way of thinking, since the substance of the mind is really Nothing, then to get to know yourself cannot mean exploring your mind. And it doesn't. A Taoist first gets to know the inner workings of his or her body. Specifically it begins with getting to know the five primary internal organs: the heart, lungs, liver, kidneys and spleen. These are really the "Gods" of our body.

How many of us has any idea what's happening inside ourselves? Not many. To follow the Way you must get to know your heart, get to know your lungs and your liver, kidneys and spleen as well. By learning to regulate the body's five major organs, you learn about yourself in a way you've probably never thought about before. But in a very real sense you are getting to know yourself.

Some theory is in order here. The five major organs provide us with a starting point to discuss the final concept necessary to understand Chi Kung. We have already discussed Tao, Chi, Jing, Shen, Yin and Yang, Tai Chi and now we get to the Five Elements.

The world and everything in it and on it is composed of these Five Elements. It is a vital part of Chinese medical theory. If I call them the Five Forces, it may simplify the meaning. Energy manifests itself as five basic forces: Fire and Water, which we have already mentioned, and Metal, Wood and Earth.

We each have these Five Forces within us. Each of our five major organs is the storehouse for one of these Five Forces. When the Five Forces are in balance we feel good, we feel healthy. When they are out of balance we get sick, or depressed or a whole host of other bad things. By learning to regulate and get in touch with our five major organs, we learn to harmonize and balance the Five Elements in our body. The principles of Yin and Yang are used to balance each of the Five Forces. For instance if our kidneys, which rule the Element of Water in our body, are too cold (Yin) we must warm them up (add Yang energy, usually from the heart, which rules the Fire Element). This makes us healthier and allows us to live longer and happier lives.

Where Do We Begin?

Between the Energy that falls to Earth from above (Taoists call this Heavenly Chi) and the Energy of the Earth itself (Earth Chi), we find the Energy of Man (Human Chi).

Chi Kung begins with the study and practice of Human Chi. For the Taoists this was a wonderful subject. When I think about it, I get a smile in my eyes. And this is a good thing. If you learn Chi Kung, then your eyes will smile too.

The Taoist approach to Human Energy will often be found to come from a totally different perspective than we are used to in the West. This is what gives Taoist Yoga its own charm and uniqueness. As I learned from my teacher, no matter how well I thought I knew what was coming next, when I actually learned a new method or technique, it always seemed to come from an unexpected angle. This is part of its beauty and mystique.

Basically Chi Kung is concerned with making us healthier and slowing down the aging process. We will use what I've called the Three-Pronged Approach. We learn to exercise our Three Treasures by regulation of the breath, regulation of the body and regulation of the mind.

I saw a need for a basic book to explain to readers from many different walks of life how to begin the practice of Taoist Yoga and Chi Kung. The best way is to find a teacher. A good teacher knows the approach must include training all Three Treasures, the Energy, the Essence and the Mind. But if this is impractical or you like to learn on your own then I've designed this book with you in mind. There are many good books on the market that describe Taoist exercises and discuss Chi Kung techniques. Most of the books tend to be either too general, too complicated or too limited to a single subject matter to be of any real use in beginning the practice on your own.

It is also possible that many sincere readers cannot find a teacher who really understands the Three Treasures of the Way and has only learned one or two of the Treasures. For instance there are those who do physical exercises and/or study martial arts but have never learned to regulate breathing or the mind. Then there are many who have learned to exercise the mind through meditation and their breath with breathing exercises but ignore their bodies.

Some of you may have taken some classes already or have studied the exercises known as Tai Chi Chuan. This book can be treated as either a refresher or a primer. The true study of Chi Kung and Taoist Yoga provides a balanced Three-Pronged Approach: Breath, Body, Mind.

Chi, the First Treasure: Regulating the Breath

When I first thought about writing this book, my initial idea was to devote the entire book to Taoist breathing techniques. Breath lies at the very core of Chi Kung which was originally the practice of breathing exercises. If you don't learn the breathing techniques, you won't get much in the way of results from the other two Treasures, the body and the mind. So the starting point for the practice is learning about breathing.

A nice thing about the breathing exercises is that they are really easy. They can be done just about anywhere, just about anytime, by just about anyone. And there are only really two basic techniques. These two techniques known as Abdominal Breathing and Reverse Breathing will be fully explained during the 100 Days of Practice. Abdominal and Reverse Breathing form the foundation for many of the other techniques we will learn in this book. Most of the moving Chi Kung we will study combines movement and breath. Many of the mental exercises utilize concentration and breath technique.

One of the unique aspects of Chi Kung is that much of the practice was developed for the old and the infirm. The most basic exercise for patients too sickly to even get out of bed is Deep Breathing. Deep Breathing stimulates Original Chi (Yuan Chi) which is often called Vital Energy. Traditional Chinese Medicine teaches that a person full of Vital Energy will enjoy good health. Chi Kung aims at stimulating Vital Energy so as to strengthen immunity to disease, increase your ability to adapt to your immediate environment and the ability to repair any internal damage.

Breathing exercises begin the practice. They are the building blocks for the attainment of physical and mental harmony, your two other Treasures.

Breathing is obviously one of the major functions that sustain our life. The Taoist breathing exercises increase our intake of oxygen. Taoists found that as children we breathe deeply, expanding our lower abdomen and diaphragm. As we age, breathing tends to get shallower and shallower. We stop using the abdominal muscles. Then we stop using the diaphragm. The lungs don't fill completely with air. Eventually the breath barely reaches the top of the lungs and stays mainly in the throat. This depletes the oxygen in our body. Taoists believe that it is the decreased intake of oxygen that is a prime cause of memory loss in the elderly.

The Taoists were also aware of a life-sustaining force in the air, aside from its major components of oxygen, nitrogen and carbon dioxide. The air also has charged particles floating in it that are called *ions*. The Taoists found that the air high up in the mountains had the greatest concentration of ions. This is a major reason many Taoists lived in the mountains of China aside from its serenity and isolation. The most important ions are *negative ions*. They help supply the electrical current within our body's cells. In our cities these ions are depleted by pollution, tightly enclosed living and working conditions, air conditioning and numerous other aspects of modern living. If our source of negative ions is depleted, we often become weak, tired or depressed.

In China machines called Chi Machines are in widespread use, especially in hospitals. They are also available in the West through New Age mail order houses and are fairly costly. These Chi Machines are really nothing more than high-end ionizers, which spew out negative ions. Ionizers are widely available in the West, where they are often combined into air cleaners with blower motors. I've even seen ionizers that work in cars by plugging them into the cigarette lighter socket. In addition to their function of supplying life-sustaining force, they also do an excellent job of cleaning the air all by themselves. Negative ions attach themselves to anything floating in the air and cause the pollutants to fall out of the air. They are excellent devices for allergy sufferers. If you can afford it, get one, two or more. Keep one in your bedroom and if you work in an office, keep another on or close to your desk.

This isn't mysticism. It is science. Ionizers were used in the American space program. Ionizers in the space capsules kept the astronauts more alert and energized. In Japan many modern office buildings use ionizers in their air filtration system. Ions found in the mountains are no better than ions produced from an ionizer. Ions are negatively charged electrons and do their job whether they are "organic" or "man-made."

Go out and get a Chi Machine, an ionizer. Even if you never practice anything in this book, the ionizer will provide you with a healthier environment and better air. It's as good as bottled mountain air. What could be better than that?

Jing, the Second Treasure: Regulating the Body

Once you learn the basic breathing techniques, the movement of the breath is used in regulating the body. This is a most un-Western concept and needs some explanation.

Movement of Chi within the body can be regulated to flow in harmony with the inhalation and exhalation of breath. One of the basic goals of Chi Kung is to learn to control the flow of Chi within the Energy Channels. There are probably places inside of you where the Energy doesn't flow smoothly. You can feel them. They are all the tight spots in your neck and shoulders, the pain in your back, the sore muscles or aching legs. Wherever it hurts or feels numb, the Chi is not flowing freely.

The exercises of the Second Treasure form the bulk of what is usually regarded as Chi Kung. These are the moving exercises. They generally combine some form of movement with breathing. Some of the movements are quite simple. Some are more complex. Many are considered to be traditional Chinese fitness exercises or calisthenics. Millions of Chinese do them every morning. I don't think it is easy to learn exercises from a book. So let's concentrate on exercises that don't involve too many movements or steps. Some Taoist moving exercises such as Tai Chi Chuan involve quite a bit of movement. It seems to me that Tai Chi Chuan, which historically is a relative newcomer, is the only well-known Chinese fitness exercise in the West. Modern forms of Tai Chi have grown increasingly complex. You can learn Tai Chi from a teacher, you can learn Tai Chi from a teacher and a book, you can probably learn it from a video and a book, but it is really hard to learn Tai Chi from just a book. Without learning correct breathing and control of the Chi flow, Tai Chi Chuan is just an elegant dance. Many Tai Chi instructors do not know Taoist Yoga; there was no one to teach them.

The exercises we will learn in our 100 Days of Practice have many interesting names and histories. There is Tao In (also called Tao Yin or Dao In) which is at least 2,500 years old. It evolved to promote health and cure certain diseases by combining regulated, controlled breathing with physical exercises. Tao In is fun and real easy to learn. In 1973, a silk scroll dated to 168 B.C. was discovered in a prince's tomb in Hunan province. The scroll depicts forty-four figures of men and women doing different Tao In exercises. Tao In exercises appear throughout the Taoist Canon which contains thousands of pages of the collected thoughts, words and practices of the Taoists spread out over hundreds of years. Tao In is very good for the lower back, legs, neck and shoulders.

A traditional Taoist fitness set we will learn is known as Baduanjin. This translates to the Eight-Sided Brocade or Eight Pieces of Brocade. It was supposedly developed by a Chinese general to keep his men fit. It is composed of eight relatively simple exercises. They are excellent for warm-ups, combining breathing with stretching. For some, the Eight Pieces of Brocade provides a complete fitness regime. It gets your Jing flowing. We will learn all eight, but not at the same time. I'll spread them out over a few weeks. They are simple and fun to do, especially if you hate to exercise.

The Muscle-Tendon Change Classic or Yi Jin Jing has a particularly interesting history. They are sort of Taoist isometric exercises combining regulation of breath with alternating tension and relaxation of the body and the extremities. If you have Abdominal Breathing down pat, these are very easy to learn. If you really hate exercising, these are for you.

Yi Jin Jing was originally created by a Buddhist monk from India who traveled to China in A.D. 527 at the request of the Chinese emperor. His name was Da Mo Sardili. He and Emperor Liang soon had a falling out and Da Mo retired to the Buddhist Temple at Shaolin. Here he found that the Chinese Buddhist monks spent most of their time meditating and ignored their bodies, and as a result many were weak and in ill-health. After spending some time in seclusion, Da Mo created the exercises known as Yi Jin Jing and taught them to the Shaolin monks. The monks found that the exercises improved their health and increased their strength and flexibility. Da Mo taught that cultivation and regulation of the body was just as important as spiritual cultivation. This was a very controversial idea among the traditionally conservative Chinese Buddhists. However, the Shaolin Temple became the center for teaching Da Mo's theories and practice. Da Mo was the founder of what has come to be known as Shaolin Kung Fu and Yi Jin Jing is its foundation, along with two other practices he also instituted known as Bone Marrow Breathing and Buddha Palm, which are too advanced for the first 100 Days of Practice. He also taught a form of meditation known in China as Charn Meditation. It was exported to Japan where it was called Zen. Da Mo was an important, enlightened human being. He is commonly called the Bodhidarma, and has legendary status in China.

In the years after Da Mo's death, his teachings were passed on to Taoist monks. The Taoists were much more open-minded than many of the conservative and highly regulated Chinese Buddhists. Yi Jin Jing, the Muscle-Tendon Change Classic, became a part of Taoist Chi Kung. The Taoists were always willing to accept any teaching or training as their own if it helped them on the Way.

The emphasis of all these physical exercises, Tao In, Baduanjin, Yi Jin Jing and many others, is not necessarily muscular development. The Taoists were much more concerned with keeping the body's connective tissue flexible.

They realized that muscular development will peak by age thirty-five no matter how much exercise you do. As you age the tendons that connect the muscles to the bone begin to tighten and shrink. It is the tightening and shrinkage of the tendons that is generally experienced as the feeling of aging. Keeping the tendons supple and filled with Chi will allow you to remain flexible well into old age.

Regulating the Organs and Fascia

Another type of connective tissue that is highly important to the practice of Chi Kung is the Fascia. It surrounds our internal organs. It's that sticky, stretchy stuff around our heart and lungs and liver and the rest of our organs.

The Fascia is used to regulate the balance of Yin Chi and Yang Chi in the organs. We use the Six Healing Sounds to cool off the five major organs and relax the body. Heat is released from the organs through the Fascia which acts like a thermostat. The Six Healing Sounds are used to get us in touch with our five major organs by the use of a simple sound combined with inhalation and exhalation of breath. The Sixth Healing Sound is directed at the Triple Warmer—the head, the chest, and the abdomen—which the Chinese recognize as a separate organ. You can't find it on any anatomy charts in the West. The Triple Warmer regulates the temperature in the head and body.

We will learn the sounds and six simple positions used to enhance them. Six Healing Sound Chi Kung is very calming and relaxing. Busy Taoists use them for stress reduction. They are excellent at night, in bed, to help you fall asleep. The Six Healing Sounds are simple and ingenious. They are a powerful form of healing Chi Kung that can literally be practiced anytime, anywhere. You'll start learning them the first week.

A different approach to the fascia will be learned toward the end of the 100 days. The fascia can be packed with Vital Energy and this energy, in turn, strengthens the internal organs. The technique we will learn is called Iron Shirt Packing Process Breathing. This is a variation on the practice of Reverse Breathing which is one of the two basic breathing techniques. By packing the fascia with Chi, the fascia is strengthened and serves to protect the internal organs. Packing Process Breathing was long a secret technique of Taoist martial artists and is the foundation of Iron Shirt Chi Kung. These martial artists learned to build an internal "iron shirt" that was impervious to the blows of their opponents. Packing Process Breathing also softens the tendons and energizes the organs and the rest of the body as well. It also helps you to grow "roots" into the ground and draw energy from the Earth.

Taoist Self-Massage Rejuvenation

Taoist Rejuvenation exercises were the first things taught to me by my teacher Mantak Chia in 1981. Over the years, I've learned dozens of techniques from Chia, other teachers, and recently from Yun Xiang Tseng, a young Chi Kung and Kung Fu Master who emigrated to the United States from mainland China a few years ago.

Self-Massage Rejuvenation consists of simple exercises and self-massage techniques that are generally aimed at specific parts of the body. There is a whole battery of techniques for massaging the face, with many different exercises for the eyes, ears, nose, teeth, gums, etc. We also learn to detoxify the organs and glands using light slapping and tapping.

A major part of Self-Massage Rejuvenation involves massaging the abdomen using the navel as the focal point. These techniques are a uniquely Taoist approach to massage.

Here we're moving Chi to different parts of the body and breaking up any blockages to the free flow of our Vital Energy. We use the mind to bring our concentration to a body part. By concentrating on a part of the body, for instance the hands and fingertips, Chi will flow to the hands and fingertips. A basic rule of Chi management is that the mind cannot push Chi, but the mind can lead the Chi. Simply put, mentally focus on a part of your body and the Chi will flow there. You then massage that spot and increase and harmonize the flow of Vital Energy there.

Self-Massage Rejuvenation revitalizes the body. It tones and beautifies the face. It gets your Chi and Jing flowing. Many of the techniques will initially seem strange to you but they are really quite logical and well thought out. They are also simple to perform and can be done by anyone. They were originally developed as longevity techniques to help ward off the effects of aging. There's something here for everyone. We will even learn the Taoist methods of swallowing air and saliva. Believe it or not, these techniques are among the most important for real success in the practice.

Throughout the 100 Days of Practice, you'll learn new Taoist Self-Massage techniques. I'll even give you one right now. Rub your two hands together, vigorously, until your palms get hot. Concentrate on Chi flowing into your palms and fingers. Once you feel heat in your palms, bring your hands to your face and gently rub your cheeks and then the sides of your nose. Rub your hands together again and then cover your eyes with your palms. The energy you feel as heat in your hands is Chi.

It is at moments like this that we can break down that mysterious barrier of what Chi is. Remember, Chi is *energy*. Heat is a form of energy. If we build up heat in our hands, then it is the same as saying we have built up Chi in our hands. If we feel that heat pass from our hands to our face when we rub it with our palms, this is the same as saying we have passed Chi from our hands to our face. If you were to rub your hands together until they were hot and then put them on someone else's face, you would be passing Chi from your hands to another person's face. There is nothing very mysterious about this. Hundreds of millions of Chinese know that Chi can be moved in your body or be sent out of your body to another person. This is an accepted truth.

As you can see, the basic concept of moving Chi is not really mysterious at all. We are talking energy here. There is nothing uniquely Chinese about energy. Everybody has energy.

Seminal and Ovarian Kung Fu: Sexual Yoga

The most powerful form of Essence in our body is our sexual energy. There is sufficient Jing in one sperm cell and one ovum to provide the Vital Energy necessary to create a life. Taoist referred to the Jing of creation as Original Essence. At conception Original Essence is converted into Original Chi.

The practice of Seminal and Ovarian Kung Fu is based on the principle of our ability to convert Sexual Essence (Jing) into Life Force Energy (Chi). We will refer to this generically as Sexual Energy (Jing Chi—which, I am aware, mixes the newer pinyin and older Wade-Giles forms of transcription, but I prefer it to Ching Chi or Jing Qi).

The Taoists realized that Sexual Energy is the only form of energy in the body that increases in force when it is activated. In other words, when you are sexually aroused, you can feel your sexual energy actually double, triple or increase even more from what it was before you were aroused. In the West we call it "getting turned on" or "horny." You know it when you feel it. Seminal and Ovarian Kung Fu make use of your Sexual Jing to transform it into Chi and provide the body with more Energy. In addition, Sexual Essence brought up the spine by a technique called Seminal or Ovarian Breathing is used to revitalize the brain.

We begin by learning to increase the production of Sexual Jing. For women this involves massaging the breasts and for men in massaging the testicles. (These exercises can't be done everywhere.) Later we will learn Seminal and Ovarian Breathing to raise the Sexual Energy to rejuvenate the brain. Finally we will learn how to draw aroused Sexual Energy into the body so that it is not lost. The theory here is a little different for men than it is for women, but the practice is pretty much the same.

Conservation of Sexual Energy is important to the practice. Men lose Jing Chi when they ejaculate, so the ability to minimize the loss of sperm is a major goal. Women do not lose Jing Chi during orgasm. As mentioned, they lose Jing Chi through menstruation. The gentle practice of Ovarian Breathing helps reduce the loss of energy from menstruation often resulting in a shorter, more regular and less troublesome period.

For both men and women, conserving Sexual Energy rather than losing it through ejaculation or menstruation provides the body with extra energy that would otherwise be lost or wasted.

This leads us to the second goal of Taoist Sexual Yoga, which is the transformation of Sexual Jing into Chi. This transformation provides the body with a great boost of energy which can be used for self-healing and revitalizing the organs and the brain. I'll explain this in more detail in the practice section.

The third goal of Seminal and Ovarian Kung Fu is to balance the body's male and female energies (Yang and Yin). This comes about as a result of following the practices (single cultivation) and also through lovemaking between a man and woman (dual cultivation) who are familiar with the techniques.

The cultivation of Sexual Energy provides a powerful, natural form of energy for the body. There is nothing sinister or illicit about it. The Taoists were honorable, virtuous people. They just had a different way of looking at life. The Taoist sexual practices are really a lot healthier and saner than most of what goes on in this world in the name of sexuality.

Shen, the Third Treasure: Regulating the Mind

Regulating the mind involves calming the mind, calming the emotions and learning to use your mind to guide and direct the flow of your Chi-Energy. This is the Chi Kung Treasure that first drew me to the practice. This is Nei Dan, or Internal Exercises as opposed to the physical exercises we have learned about, which are called *Wei Dan*.

The inner world of the Taoists was filled with many unique approaches to how we are capable of using our minds. This part of Chi Kung is fun. It is also, in many ways, the most profound part of the practice.

We will begin by learning a simple technique to calm down and focus our mind. We will put our attention on our breath and learn to concentrate on specific points within our bodies. It is important to calm our mind when doing Internal Chi Kung. If the mind is not calmed down, it is easily distracted, and it is filled with runaway thoughts and real concentration is impossible.

A major goal of Tao Masters was the silencing of the mind. The exercises you will learn will assist you to begin working on achieving this goal. We will not expect miracles. Silencing all the thought processes of the mind usually requires a real effort of will power applied over a substantial period of time.

One reward for calming down the mind is our increased ability to concentrate. This in turn results in our becoming able to learn techniques to focus inside of ourselves and get in touch with our organs. This is really new territory for the Western mind. How do you get in touch with your internal organs? Well, I've already mentioned the Six Healing Sounds as one method. Another is the marvelous technique called the Inner Smile. The Inner Smile was a true Taoist secret. Who but the Taoist could ever come up with a basic practice that uses smiling energy?

The Taoists tended to be happy individuals. They are often pictured with smiling, inscrutable eyes. These Taoists had a secret technique to develop and maintain those smiling eyes, the secret was the practice of the Inner Smile. First they learned to smile into their eyes, and then they learned to turn this smile inward and direct it into the organs, into the digestive system, into the brain and spine and eventually into the whole body. The benefits of the Inner Smile are almost too many to mention. First, it continues the work of calming and focusing the mind. The Inner Smile along with the Six Healing Sounds are the two basic Taoist practices for stress control. Smiling energy has great healing potential. The Inner Smile helps to release trapped negative energy and replace it with happy, positive energy. This may sound silly, but so much of the Taoist practices have their own unique logic to them. It's just that we were never taught to think along Taoist lines. Smiling into an organ and filling it with happy, loving energy, as a calming and self-healing technique, really makes perfect sense. My teacher never tired of saying that you really cannot love somebody else until you learn to love yourself. But he was never talking about narcissistic self-love, or worship of the unruly ego. No. He literally meant to learn to love yourself from the inside out. After a while at the practice, the smile begins to radiate from inside of you. Other people will sense your smiling energy and react favorably to it. A real smile can often work "miracles." A real smile that comes from deep within you is like a ray of sunshine on a cloudy day. So we will learn, as the I Ching says, to "Be not sad, be like the Sun at Midday."

Each of the five major organs corresponds with one of the Five Elements. By learning to direct smiling energy into each of the five major organs, we begin the process of balancing the Five Elements inside of our body. This has a direct effect on our emotional state.

The process works like this: the organs control the balance of the Elements inside of us. These Elements control our emotional state. By smiling into our organs, we get them to calm down, relax and function more efficiently and most importantly convert negative emotions into positive emotions. This in turn helps to balance the Five Elements. Balancing the Five Elements neutralizes negative emotions resulting in a more positive emotional state.

Western psychology looks almost exclusively at the brain as the control center of our emotions. The Taoists have known for thousands of years that our internal organs play a key role as well. Too many of us are no more aware of what is going on inside ourselves than we are of what goes on inside of our cars or computers. But doesn't it make sense that to keep ourselves healthy we should be aware of our major organs and keep them happy and healthy by smiling into them and thanking them for keeping us alive? It does to the Taoists.

The final technique we will learn for regulating the mind is known as Opening the Microcosmic Orbit. This involves using the mind to direct the flow of Chi in our two major Energy Meridians. The first is the Governor Channel which runs from just below the tip of the spine at the perineum, up the backbone and neck and over the top of the head, ending in the roof of the mouth. The Functional Channel runs from the tip of your tongue, down through the throat, continuing down the middle of your body, past the navel, through the lower abdomen and sexual organs and ends in the perineum, which is located between the sexual organs and the anus in both men and women.

You might have noticed that the Functional Channel ends in the perineum, the same spot where the Governor Channel begins. When these two Channels are connected, they are called The Microcosmic Orbit. Chi runs in a continuous circuit up the back, over the head and down the front of the body until it circles around past the genitals and back up the spine. The Microcosmic Orbit was once a highly secret technique. Today it is done every day by millions of Chinese.

Our Original Chi flowed unobstructed in the Microcosmic Orbit when we were children. Over the years, blockages appear. They can be caused by emotional trauma, or injury, poor posture, bad eating habits, bad breathing habits and a whole host of other causes. The result is that Energy does not flow through the entire Microcosmic Orbit any longer, it only flows through parts of the Governor and Functional Channel. We no longer feel the continuous flow of energy, instead we feel disconnected, disjointed, pain, numbness and fatigue. The Opening of the Microcosmic Orbit does just that, it opens up the blockages and allows the Chi to once again flow smoothly.

We will learn to Open the Microcosmic Orbit gradually. It can be learned from a book if we take each step slowly and practice. By the end of 100 Days of Practice your Orbit should be open. For some of you it will spring open spontaneously, others will have to put a lot of effort into it. Once your Orbit is open, you will feel like a new person. But if you don't practice, you will get no results.

The mind is used to guide the Chi up the Governor Channel and down the Functional Channel in the Microcosmic Orbit. This is not an easy concept for many Westerners. But it really is simple. You *cannot* push Chi with your mind. You *can* lead Chi with your thoughts. This is why it is important to start the practice of Regulating the Mind by learning to concentrate on specific spots in our body. We are learning to direct our mind and our thoughts inside of ourselves, something you've probably never learned before. Chi will follow your point of concentration. That is one of the ways that Chi works. At the start of the practice, it often feels like all you are doing is exercising your imagination. But with a little practice you will begin to feel warm Energy moving inside you. Usually you feel it first behind the navel. The practice is also known as the Warm Current Method. Opening the Microcosmic Orbit is a crucial part of Taoist health, sexuality, rejuvenation and longevity practice. Once it is open, you can take it with you everywhere, and it just might become one of your greatest possessions.

道

part two

道 *The*
Practice

100 Days to Better Health, Good Sex & Long Life

THE TAOISTS TAUGHT THAT THE length of time necessary to give birth to the Immortal Fetus was one hundred days. This Immortal Fetus would then require many years of care and nurturing before it was capable of actually leaving the body and existing independently. In practical terms, one hundred days was the amount of time necessary to establish a firm foundation in the practice of Taoist Yoga. By the end of one hundred days you should have begun to feel warmth in the lower abdomen.

One hundred days breaks down to just a bit over fourteen weeks, about a week longer than three months. That makes for a fourteen-week program of authentic Taoist practices, using a three-pronged approach: regulating the breath, body and mind. We begin right away with the care and nurturing of the Three Treasures: Chi, Jing and Shen (Energy, Essence and Mind).

I will attempt to explain each exercise or technique in sufficient detail so that you can practice on your own without a teacher present. I'll try to anticipate your questions so there is no confusion on just how to do it right. Most of the training will build upon itself week by week, month by month, as we slowly develop a repertoire of techniques. As we work through the one hundred days, new practices and techniques will be introduced that previously you were not ready for.

It is important to take things slowly and master each step. That is one of the nice aspects of learning from this book. We can work at a leisurely pace and not hurry ahead to the next step before we're ready. This is an important factor. In our busy lives, those of us who've had the time or opportunity to take a workshop on Taoist Yoga or Chi Kung will have a lot of information thrown at us in a short period of time. This often results in the student leaving the class with the last thing learned most impressed upon his or her mind, which is usually the most advanced practice taught at the seminar. As a result, the more basic practices are often overlooked.

So, learning Chi Kung from this book can be very rewarding if you pay attention to the text, and practice every day. We're not looking for a big commitment here. Give it at least fifteen minutes a day. Soon you'll probably want to do more, but fifteen minutes is all I ask. Of course when you are first reading about and learning a technique, it may take a little more time to absorb the lesson. But, in general, to begin the practice does not require a large time commitment.

Don't expect miracles at the beginning of the practice. The inner power of Taoist Yoga must be built on a firm foundation. You will probably not be able to shoot beams of Chi across the room for a while yet. This book is about learning to control Chi. It takes time and effort to learn. That's why it's called Chi KUNG. Before you can control Chi outside of yourself, you must be able to control it inside of yourself. As Master Chia always said, "If you do it, you get it. If you don't do it, you don't get it."

You are responsible for your own progress. You are your own master and you will decide for yourself how far you will progress in your practice as well as in your life. In Chi Kung there are no gurus, only teachers. A highly proficient teacher is known as a Master. There is no master-servant relationship indicated or implied between the teacher and the student. A Tao Master respects each person's autonomy. Never give up your will or common sense to anybody.

Remember, *you* are your own Master.

Preliminary Instructions

The most important preliminary instruction is to practice every day. Many teachers and some of the literature stress practicing at the same time every day. My experience is that it's nice if you can do this, but it's all right if you can't.

You should find a space with good lighting and ventilation, neither too hot nor too cold. Exercising outside is always preferred but is not often practical, especially in cold climates. In rainy, foggy or windy weather, exercise indoors. It is better if your exercises are done in a quiet place. Light music in the background is acceptable but really not necessary. Actually any space you have available to do the practices is acceptable. What is most important is daily exercise. A beautiful park-like setting with a small river running through it, or a mountain peak can certainly enhance your experience, but the bottom line is to make do with what is available to you. Taoists are eminently practical people. They make the best use of what is available to them.

Keep your mind peaceful and at ease during the physical exercises. Stay calm and relaxed. Your posture and movements should be correct. Read the instructions for each exercise carefully. Reread the instructions; there may well be a step or a hint that you missed the first time around. Doing an exercise improperly can prevent your making progress with your training.

Wear loose-fitting clothing during the exercises. No special uniform is required. Cotton was the Taoist fabric of choice and a raw silk Kung Fu outfit is nice too, but neither are necessary. Take off any jewelry that interferes when you practice. Because Chi Kung is so interrelated with breathing, tight, constricting clothes can impede the breathing process. For men, boxer shorts are preferable to briefs, because they allow the testicles to hang naturally without binding them up; this is important to the practice. Women should avoid a tight brassiere, but the choice to wear one or not depends on how comfortable you are. If you feel that you need it or want it, then wear it.

Don't eat before you practice in the morning; practicing with a full stomach affects your digestion and tends to make you slow, sluggish, and tired. Likewise, don't practice when you are hungry. It's too difficult to concentrate. As far as diet is concerned, cut down on greasy food and sweets. Meat is permitted but a heavy diet of steaks and chops should be tempered. These, too, tend to slow you down. Overall, use common sense. Don't change your lifestyle and your eating habits all at once. You will only fail. Make changes gradually. Usually when you are ready to make a change, your body will tell you. The Taoist practices are designed to get you in better touch with your body and eventually you will be more sensitive to its needs. You will make any changes to your diet when and if you're ready to. You are your own master.

Many Taoist sects were totally vegetarian. Many were not. Some ate no grains or rice. Some ate almost nothing but rice. Some favored simple fare, others elaborate, creative cooking. Some followed Five Element cooking by balancing the five flavors: sweet, sour, salty, bitter and pungent (spicy). There is no fixed rule. Taoists are flexible. Eat what you want. If your conscience tells you to stop or if you feel that your eating habits are negatively affecting your life, then stop and make some changes.

Smoking, of course, is frowned upon. If you are completely hooked, the deep breathing exercises can help you to cut down. When you smoke a cigarette, usually you will take a longer inhalation than your normal breath. Often it is the long inhalation which is the most pleasurable part of smoking. The breathing exercises, with their emphasis on long, slow breathing, should help to control the craving. Actually these practices are very helpful if you want to stop smoking. But don't expect miracles. When you are ready and willing to stop smoking, you will. It's all a question of what's really important to you. Since you now know what your greatest possession is, it is really time to consider stopping. Those things will kill you.

Excessive alcohol should be avoided, although a daily glass of wine is recommended in some of the ancient literature found in the Taoist Canon. One glass helps you to relax. More than one helps you to get drunk.

The use of narcotic drugs is, naturally, forbidden. Some ancient Taoists did take various herbs, herbal remedies and liquid elixirs. This was also part of their search for the pill of immortality and was known as "external elixir alchemy." Some of these remedies were toxic, containing mercury, arsenic, and cinnabar. No known pill of immortality was ever discovered. Many were useful for a variety of other reasons. Some of the formulas still exist, but you would need a Chinese apothecary (that can be found in the Chinatown section of any major city) to get the ingredients. Chinese pharmacies sell pills that are used to balance the energy of individual organs. These are useful in balancing the Five Elements but are by no means absolutely necessary to the practice. Without a knowledgeable teacher around, ingesting anything that is going to change your body chemistry is always questionable. Modern Western vitamin and herbal dietary supplements basically serve the same purpose as the Chinese remedies, which is to keep us healthy, energized, and mentally fit.

Men should try to decrease the number of times they ejaculate. The body expends a tremendous amount of energy creating sperm cells. When the scrotum is full, the body cuts back on sperm production and this energy is conserved for other bodily functions. The loss of sperm causes the body's sperm factories to move into high gear. Continual drainage of sperm will keep these factories working full time, depleting your Chi and Jing. Note that I am not advocating cutting back on sex. Just ejaculate less often. This is especially true for men after forty. The Taoist secrets of seminal retention were often used as rejuvenation methods for older men. Keeping the Sexual Essence within, rather than mindlessly wasting it, is among the most potent of all the Taoist health, rejuvenation, and longevity practices. The emphasis of lovemaking shifts away from the quick orgasm toward sustained ability to maintain an erection. Women gain as well from longer, slower sex, where the goal is not merely to bring their partner to orgasm, but rather for both partners to sustain their pleasure. The balance of Yin and Yang between you and your partner should harmonize. In other words, your sex life should take a dramatic turn for the better.

On the other hand, celibacy works too, at least for the 100 Days of Practice; after that the Taoists believe that enforced celibacy will make you crazy or neurotic. The Taoists use sexuality to enhance the Life Force Energy, not to deplete it. This is really a new concept to the West, but the Taoist healing love techniques go back thousands of years to the time of the Yellow Emperor, one of the three "founders" of Chinese civilization.

Also, it's important not to practice with a full bladder. It disturbs your concentration if you try to hold in the urine as you exercise. It's all right to relieve yourself in the middle of a session. Just stop and go to the toilet. Don't be embarrassed if you belch or pass wind. Sometimes these things happen as we practice. Pay it no mind.

Taoists had varying beliefs about the best time to practice. In the evening, the hours between 11 P.M. and 1 A.M. are most highly recommended, and between 5 P.M. and 7 P.M. are also acceptable. In the morning, the hours of 5 A.M. to 7 A.M. are best, and 11 A.M. to 1 P.M. are all right. Exercising in the afternoon, between the hours of 1 P.M. to 3 P.M., is *not* recommended. The reasons for these rules are complicated and are based on the complex Chinese calendar and astrology. I personally don't place too much stress on them and put them here mainly for informational purposes. Try following them if you wish and see if they help your practice. If they don't, ignore them.

Again, the most important preliminary instruction is to practice every day for at least fifteen minutes. You can practice once a day, twice a day or more often than that. You can practice for hours if you wish. But practicing every day is the most important thing. If you are sick, don't do anything that tires you out or gets you overheated, but you can always do breathing exercises.

At last, we're now ready to begin the first week of practice.

THE MOST BASIC OF ALL Chi Kung exercises is breathing. In our first week of training we will learn to pay attention to and monitor our own natural breathing process. We will also learn the basic rules of Chi Kung Deep Breathing.

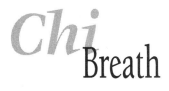

The primary meaning of Chi is breath. Before we leap off into any other method of breath regulation, it is important for us to be aware of how we breathe. Breathing is something that we all do naturally. There is no reason to even have to think about it. Nobody suffocates from forgetting to breathe. It is instinctual.

Very few of us receive instructions on how to breathe. If you're a singer or a swimmer, you may have received some training, but most of us go through life without thinking about breathing unless we get sick or injured and our breathing is affected.

So right now, I want you to listen to yourself breathe. Don't try and regulate it or alter its pattern in any way. Just pay attention to the way you normally breathe for about a minute. Make some written or mental notes about what you observe.

First of all, could you hear yourself breathing? Most of us can hear ourselves breathe. Was your breathing loud or quiet? Was it rough or smooth? If someone was standing next to you could they hear you breathe? Was your breathing shallow, into the upper part of the chest only or was it deeper into the chest? Did your diaphragm move as you inhaled and exhaled? Could you see your chest rise and fall with each breath? Did you see your belly expand

and contract with each breath? Was your breathing rapid or slow? Was it regular or irregular? Was your inhalation the same length as your exhalation? Did you pause between breaths? Did you breathe through your nose or your mouth? Just listen and sense what is going on with each breath. It might surprise you. Listen to yourself breathe again for about a minute.

The goal of this week's breathing exercises is to make you aware of your natural way of breathing and lead you to breathe in a slow and quiet manner. A Chi Kung breath should be slow, deep, even and silent. But this takes training and that's why you're here.

Breathe through your nose unless otherwise instructed. You can practice breathing anytime or anywhere. A proper breath should be gentle and quiet. This requires a calm mind. In this week's Regulation of the Mind exercise, we will do a structured practice combining calming the mind and monitoring and regulating the breath. All the exercises are interrelated. There are few "pure" exercises that only affect one of the Three Treasures. Breathing affects both the body and the mind.

Breath and mind are much more connected than most of us realize. Our emotional state often dictates the manner in which we breathe. When we're angry, we take short rapid breaths into the stomach. When we're anxious, we also take short, quick breaths but we only breathe into the upper chest. When we're happy, we take longer, slower, deeper breaths. Controlling the breath in turn helps to control the Emotional Mind, which the Taoist called the Hsin Mind.

For the first three days of this week, practice breathing the way you normally do. Just be aware of yourself breathing. You can practice when you first get out of bed. It helps to wake you up and clear your head. Just monitor your breathing for a few minutes. You can also do this at any time of the day or evening. If you do it as you lie down in bed at night, it will relax you and help you to sleep.

By the fourth day of the week, I want you to take a little more conscious control of the breathing process. The breathing we do next is preparation for Abdominal Breathing which you will begin learning next week. Breathe longer and deeper. Take in more air, which means you bring more oxygen into your system. Breathe evenly. The length of your inhalation should match the length of your exhalation. Do not pause between breaths or between inhalation and exhalation. Just continue breathing as smoothly and quietly as you can.

Try to breathe down to the diaphragm, which is at the bottom of the lungs. Instead of expanding your chest or belly as you inhale, let the breath push down on your diaphragm. Relax your chest as you inhale. Don't hold the muscles tight. Relax your chest and let the entering air push down on your diaphragm. Your chest or belly shouldn't rise as much as it did at the start of the week. Don't use force. Breathe calmly. When you exhale, slowly relax the diaphragm. This is the beginning of Deep Breathing.

You can count your breaths as an aid to making the breath even, so that the length of an inhalation matches the length of an exhalation. A four-count inhalation and four-count exhalation is excellent for beginners. With each inhalation count: one, two, three, four. Then exhale: one, two three, four. Do this for five to ten minutes each day for the rest of the week. Deep Breathing is excellent first thing in the morning. It gets your Chi flowing. It also is beneficial any time of day. It helps wake you up if you're tired. It gets more oxygen into your system. It is a simple exercise that can be done any time, anywhere. If you do it properly, without making a racket each time you breathe, no one will even know you're exercising.

Deep Breathing is a good habit to get yourself into. At the beginning, it might not be easy. For many of us, our diaphragm might be stiff and inflexible. It might feel sore for a few days as you start to work it again.

Deep Breathing is the most basic of all Chi Kung exercises. In China it is taught to convalescents who are bedridden. They are taught to breathe normally through the nose—regularly, slowly, evenly, and quietly. With each inhalation they say the word "calm" silently to themselves and with each exhalation, the word "relaxed." It can be used to soothe the entire body. If you are incapable of any other physical exercise, Deep Breathing can be performed three or four times a day for up to 20 to 30 minutes at a time. You can also relax different parts of your body as you do the breathing. Begin with the head, then the arms, hands, chest, abdomen, back, small of the back, buttocks, legs and feet. Relax all your muscles. Next concentrate on relaxing the blood vessels, nerves and internal organs. This exercise can be used by anyone for relaxation and stress reduction. Just inhale and silently say "calm" and then exhale silently saying "relaxed."

Regulating the Breath: Week One

1. Days One through Three: Breath normally and pay attention to your breathing pattern for 5 to 10 minutes daily. You can always do more if you're so inclined. This basically holds true for all the exercises.

2. Days Four through Seven: Deep Breathing—Breathe through the nose—long, slow, even, quiet breaths. Try to breathe into the

diaphragm. Relax the chest. It doesn't rise and fall as much. Breathe to a count of four. Do five to ten minutes daily.

3. Supplementary Exercise: The Relaxing Breath—Inhale silently saying "calm." Exhale silently saying "relaxed." This can also be used to relax a different body part as you breathe, any time. It's good for relaxation, stress reduction, and when recovering from an illness.

Jing Body

SOME PEOPLE GET UP IN the morning and want to do vigorous physical exercise; others hate to get out of bed and are just glad they can find their way to the bathroom. Since I can't be there to make up a personal program just for you, I have to include exercises and practices that satisfy the extremes of the two types of people mentioned above as well as everyone in between. If you are physically active and regularly exercise, continue to do vigorous exercise as well as the exercises you find here.

There is a lot to learn in this first week. The exercises don't take a long time to actually perform. But first you should be sure that you are getting them right. Read the instructions carefully, then read them again, frequently. Beginning the Taoist practices is a wonderful time. You will be learning new and wondrous information about yourself and how you function. Treat it like the beginning of an adventure.

So a good place to begin our Taoist adventure is in bed when you get up and greet the day. If you're a procrastinator and getting up in the morning (or whenever you get up) is difficult, this is a good time to begin your breathing exercises. For the first three days, just listen to and monitor your breathing. This will help to get you focused and get your Chi flowing. By the fourth day, do Deep Breathing with long, slow breaths and expansion of the diaphragm just described in Week One – Regulating the Breath. As you breathe into your diaphragm, the increased flow of oxygen into your lungs will help to stimulate the blood flow and give you a little more energy. It will help to get yourself out of bed. At first you may not feel the Deep Breath, as your body begins its waking process. But after a few breaths you will begin to feel the increased pressure on your diaphragm. Deep Breathing, using the diaphragm, exercises and strengthens your midsection as well as your entire upper body.

I've told you quite a bit about inhaling air, but so far I haven't discussed exhaling in any great detail. The Taoists practiced six specific methods of exhaling breath. These are known as the Six Healing Sounds. It's time to learn the first one.

The First Healing Sound: The Lung Sound

Since we are learning about breathing, it is appropriate that the first Healing Sound we learn is the Lung Sound. As I first learned the Healing Sounds, they were taught in a specific order and the Lung Sound was the first sound in the series. To better appreciate the Healing Sounds, it is helpful to understand what each sound is intended to achieve and how it fits into the big picture of our 100 Days of Practice.

I previously mentioned that the Healing Sound helps to release heat from the organs through the fascia which surrounds each organ and regulates its temperature. When we are tense or stressed out, the fascia tends to contract and stick to the organ. This prevents the fascia from properly doing its job. Insufficient heat is released from the organ resulting in a build-up of heat and toxins. This has a direct effect on our health and our emotions.

Modern-day society has helped to create lifestyles for many of us that are filled with physical and emotional stress. We live in overcrowded cities, with pollution, noise and traffic. We eat too much junk food and take in too many chemical additives. We are often anxious or lonely. We sit too much and counter this with sudden vigorous exercise. All of this physical and emotional stress leads to tension that we feel in our bodies. This tension blocks the free flow of Chi-Energy in our body, one result of which is the constriction of the fascia around our major organs and the overheating of the organs. Continued overheating of an organ causes it to harden and contract. Its ability to function properly is inhibited and eventually, if not remedied, will result in illness.

An overheated organ affects the balance of the Five Elements. Each of the five major organs controls one of these Five Elements. The lungs control the Metal Element. Metal can have a positive or negative effect on our body and our state of mind. Overheated lungs would have a negative effect on the Metal Element. This in turn affects other organs. But the Taoists discovered that negative elements or forces also create and control negative emotions. The negative emotions resulting from overheated, stressed lungs are sadness, grief and depression.

The Healing Sound for the Lung begins the process of releasing negative emotions by releasing heat from the lung. This might all sound like lunacy, but these practices were developed thousands of years ago by true Tao Masters and are well known in the Taoist Canon. If done diligently, they really work.

Sound is actually a vibration. Each sound vibrates at a particular frequency. The Tao Masters long ago discovered that a healthy organ vibrates at a particular frequency. Each of the Six Healing Sounds vibrates at one of the six correct frequencies necessary to keep all of the five major organs and the Triple Warmer in optimal condition to prevent and alleviate sickness.

The really good thing about all this is that the Healing Sounds are ridiculously easy to do. The Healing Sound for the lungs is S-S-S-S-S-S-S-S. Like a soft lazy snake. What could be easier than that?

The sound is made only upon exhalation. The sound by itself will have a positive effect on the body. However, there are specific movements designed to enhance the Healing Sounds. We call them Healing Sounds Chi Kung. Here is the first one.

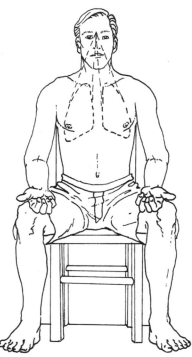

1. This exercise is done sitting on a chair. Your hands rest in your lap with the palms facing upward. Keep your eyes open. Don't do this exercise while driving.

2. Place your awareness on your lungs. Try to feel them inside of you. Your lungs are under your rib cage in your chest. If you are unsure of their exact location, don't worry. If you can sense nothing, just visualize them inside you.

3. Take a deep breath with a four-count inhalation. For the first three days just take a four-count breath without using the diaphragm. After that, expand your diaphragm as you inhale, keeping your chest relaxed.

4. As you inhale, raise your hands, palms upward, in front of your body. When they reach eye level, you must rotate the palms as you continue to raise them above your head, so they remain facing upward. Keep the elbows rounded.

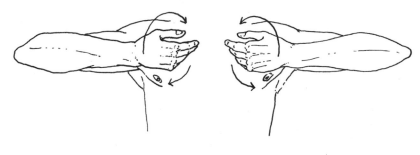

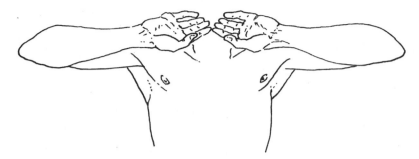

5. Your eyes follow your hands as you raise them above your head.

6. Close your jaws so that the teeth meet gently. Your lips should be slightly open and the corners of your mouth should be somewhat drawn back as you exhale. The tip of your tongue should be touching your lower gums just below your bottom front teeth. Allow your escaping breath to exit between your teeth.

7. As you exhale, very gently make the sound S-S-S-S-S-S-S-S to a count of four. Do it subvocally as you become more experienced. By this I mean that initially the sound should be barely audible. When it is subvocal it is inaudible even though you are still making the sound. If you do it silently enough, eventually the sound seems to vibrate directly in your lungs.

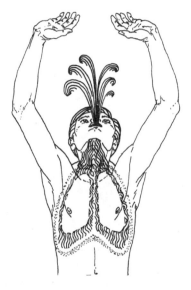

8. As you exhale and make the S-S-S-S-S-S-S sound, try to visualize and feel the fascia known as the pleura which surrounds the lungs like a sack.

9. As you exhale, sense or feel heat radiating out of your pleura.

10. Visualize your lungs bathed in a metallic white light. Eject any sick energy, sadness, sorrow or grief. Just sense or imagine them leaving along with the excess heat from the lungs as you exhale.

11. When you have finished exhaling, slowly lower your palms back to your lap.

12. Rest and take one or two ordinary breaths.

13. Take another deep breath. Repeat at least three times at each session.

At first don't worry about whether you feel anything inside. Better yet, don't worry at all. Get used to the exercise. Do it as best you can. The sound itself is healing. By the end of Week One your lungs will feel better. If you are not good at visualizing, that's all right. Visualizing is a skill that comes easily to some and mystifies others. If you can't visualize then just try to sense your lungs with a sack surrounding them. Please use your imagination to see your lungs surrounded by a white metallic light. This is the color of the Metal Element. The active use of the imagination as an aid to performing the exercises is encouraged. In time what you thought was just imagination will become real.

The S-S-S-S-S-S-S-S sound works whether you do the Chi Kung movement or not. You can do them any time if you're just making the sound. Above, I cautioned against doing the exercise while driving. This is for your own safety. The full exercise involves use of senses which could take your mind off of the road. However, feel perfectly free to make the sound S-S-S-S-S-S-S-S as you exhale while driving. Just don't do any of the hand movements, visualizing or inner sensing. Just make the sound.

Make the S-S-S-S-S-S-S-S sound at least three times every day. You can do it as many times as you like; you really can't do too many. The recommended number is between three and six at each session, but this number actually applies when you are practicing more than one Healing Sound, and right now you only know one. So practice the Lung Healing Sound Chi Kung this week. You don't have to do it every time you do a breathing exercise, but make sure you do it at least three times every day.

Regulating the Body: Taoist Self-Massage Rejuvenation

Taoist Self-Massage Rejuvenation uses Chi to strengthen and rejuvenate the sense organs such as the eyes, ears, nose, tongue, teeth and skin as well as the internal organs. It works by clearing blockages from the Energy Channels or Meridians of the sense and internal organs.

Over the years I've learned so many of these techniques that I couldn't begin to get them all into a book like this. So you'll learn those that are most appropriate, and my personal favorites. Some of these techniques are unusual or even amusing. Over time they work to improve your complexion, vision, hearing, sense of smell, digestion, and they keep your teeth and gums healthy as well as improve your stamina. There are techniques for every part of the body you could ever imagine. None of these techniques is really strenuous and most are not like traditional exercises at all.

The first Self-Massage technique I've already taught you. Rub your hands together until the skin of your palms gets hot. Your left and right hand each contain the starting point for six of the body's major Energy Meridians. This adds up to a total of twelve of the body's thirty-two major Channels. Rubbing your hands together until the surface gets hot stimulates these twelve Meridians and affects your whole body.

Rubbing the Hands Together to Gather Chi

1. Spread each elbow out to its respective side.

2. Bend elbows and bring both hands together a few inches in front of the mid-section of your body between the navel and your solar plexus (at the bottom center of your front rib cage).

3. Your fingertips should be facing forward and each finger should be touching its respective neighbor or neighbors—fingers are held together, including thumb, and not loosely apart.

4. Rub the two hands together vigorously. The direction of the rubbing is forward and back, not up and down or sideways or a circular motion. The left hand and fingertips move forward as the right hand moves back and then the right hand moves forward as the left hand moves back.

5. Concentrate on your hands. Imagine that Chi is flowing to your hands. Imagine that your fingers and palms are getting hot.

6. Within a short period of time, the friction from rubbing the palms together should first cause them to become warm and then become hot. Hot is best. If your hands are dry, it is sometimes hard to get the necessary friction. In that case just continue rubbing your hands a little longer, hold your breath and concentrate on your fingertips heating up. You will find that sometimes the heat comes right up and sometimes you really have to work at it. You'll also find that sometimes you can barely get your palms to warm up at all. This is all part of the pattern of Chi flow through the body and why the Chinese devised good times and bad times to exercise. See if you can discern any patterns of Chi flow within yourself. You can record your observations in a notebook.

7. Once your hands become hot, realize that this heat is Chi. Use your imagination to gather Chi into both hands. Use your mind to direct the energy into your palms and fingertips.

Rubbing the Nose

In this first week of practice we are concentrating on exercise involving breath. Our nose serves a vital function in the breathing process. Taoists always inhale and exhale through the nose unless they are doing one of the Six Healing Sounds. When doing a Healing Sound (so far I've only taught you the Lung Sound: S-S-S-S-S-S-S) you inhale through the nose and exhale through the mouth.

The nose has three Energy Meridians running through it. The Governor Channel, one of our two main channels (which begins at the perineum and runs up the spine and neck, over the top of our head, down the nose and ends in the roof of the mouth), runs right down the middle and on both sides of the nose. The other two channels are for the large intestines and the stomach.

The nose serves three basic functions:

1. The intake and exhalation of air.

2. Cleaning and filtering the air to prevent dirt from reaching the lungs.

3. Regulating the temperature of the air. This is especially important in cold weather; the nose helps to warm the air before it reaches the lungs.

If you have poor circulation in the nose, its temperature regulating function goes awry, allowing extreme temperatures to reach the lungs. This makes us susceptible to upper respiratory illnesses and cold viruses. People who do the Taoist practices get far fewer colds than people who do not. In the fifteen years I've known him, I never once saw Mantak Chia with a cold.

Rubbing the nose strengthens the temperature regulator, stimulates the three Meridians and increases hormonal secretion as well as toning the flesh and beautifying the skin.

Rubbing the Sides of the Nose

1. Begin by rubbing the hands together to gather the Chi.

2. When the hands get hot bring them to the side of your nose with the index finger at the bottom (thumbs are spread out of the way) and the middle finger above it on the fleshy part of the nose.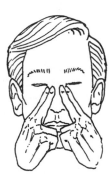

3. Simultaneously massage both sides of the nose with your index and middle fingers moving up and down together until your nose feels warm. Rub a minimum of 9 times and a maximum of 36.

4. Use very little force initially; the nose is a sensitive and delicate area.

This exercise is excellent to help you get up in the morning, especially on cold winter mornings. Initially you might find that your nose is stiff and is tender to the rubbing. Be gentle. In time the cartilage, connective tissue and muscles will all relax and you will feel all sorts of movement under your fingertips as you massage, especially at the point where your nasal bone ends and the cartilage, which gives the nose shape, begins.

Up to now, Western exercise has neglected the nose. A massaged nose not only has all the benefits already mentioned but it also helps to relax tension in the face. When you begin rubbing your nose, you will soon realize how tight and full of tension it is. Rubbing the sides of the nose breaks up blockages and gets the Chi and blood flowing into the middle of your face, and from there it spreads out into the rest of your face.

Rubbing the Bridge of the Nose

The bridge of the nose is located at the top of the nose between the two eyes.

1. Rub hands together until they are hot. If you are continuing from above, Rubbing the Sides of the Nose, just rub your hands together briefly.

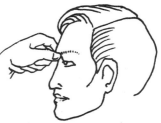

2. Use only the thumb and index finger of one hand. The choice of left or right hand is up to you.

3. Massage the bridge of the nose on the left and right side of the nose, near the inner corner of the eyes, between the thumb and index finger.

4. Pinch down on either side of the bridge, between the two fingers, repeatedly. Taoists call this point the Yin Tang.

5. As you massage and pinch, inhale slowly to a count of four and imagine that you are breathing in clean, rejuvenating air. Exhale slowly through your nose, to count of four and imagine that you are exhaling old, weak or sickly air. The cleansing inhalation loosens up dirt and impurities in the lungs which are expelled with a slow 4-count exhalation.

This exercise is effective for clearing blocked sinuses. It helps to detoxify the respiratory system and make you feel better. Active use of the imagination really helps to make these exercises work. You are learning new ways to look at yourself and treat your body. If you believe in the exercises, they work. At the beginning of undertaking this 100 Days of Practice, belief in what you're doing is a helpful mindset. After you've spent a few weeks doing the program, then evaluate for yourself whether you feel that you've made any progress. If not, a little bit of skepticism might be appropriate. If you start out with a positive attitude and do the exercises every day you should feel results within the first few weeks if not sooner.

Massaging the Lower Nose

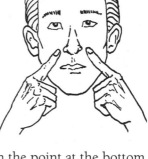

There are three points at the bottom of the nose that are useful in Self-Massage Rejuvenation, when properly activated. Two of the points are at the bottom of and just to the outside of each nostril. In Chinese they are known as the Yingxiang points. The third point, the Yen Chong, is at the bottom center of the nose, right above the middle of your lips.

1. Using the left and right index fingers, press on the point at the bottom of each nostril, the Yingxiang, just to the outside of the nostril where you should find a slight indentation.

2. Press in with the index finger on each side and make small circular movements with the fingertip as you press for 5 to 10 seconds.

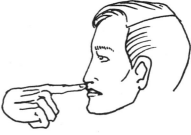

3. With either the left or right index finger press hard on the spot at the very bottom of the nose, the Yen Chong, between and below the two nostrils, and again make small circular movements with the fingertip as you press for 5 to 10 seconds.

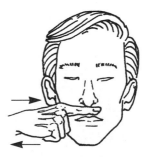

4. Take either index finger and place it at a right angle (toward the side of your cheek) to the bottom of your nose. Rub back and forth as vigorously as is comfortable between 9 and 36 times.

This exercise or any part of it is good for your sinuses and stuffy, runny noses and really helps to get your "motor running" in the morning. The three points, especially the central Yen Chong, are used in the martial arts to help revive someone who has been knocked unconscious.

Rubbing the Face

To finish this set of nasal massages, we will learn to Rub the Face. There are literally dozens of very specific techniques for massaging the face. We will learn a simple, generic method.

1. Rub the hands together until hot.

2. Rub the hands up and down on your cheeks until your hands begin to cool.

3. Rub hands together again and rub all over face and forehead.

4. Feel the heat from your hands passing into the skin of your face and forehead.

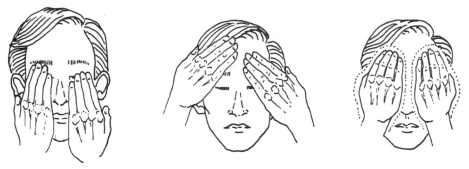

5. Rub hands together again and cover right and left eyes with a cupped palm. Absorb the heat into both eyes for at least 10 seconds.

During any of these exercises you can try doing the following if you're feeling tense or stressed. When you inhale say to yourself "calm" and when you exhale say to yourself "relaxed." How can you be tense when you're calm and relaxed?

Slapping the Chest

The final Self-Massage Rejuvenation technique for this week is called Slapping the Chest. Literally that is what we do. Slapping helps to clean out mucous and detoxify the lungs.

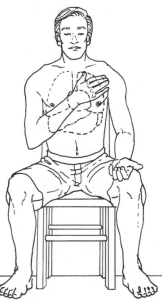

1. Rub hands together until hot.

2. Using your right palm, slap up and down the chest over the left lung. Slap only as hard as is comfortable. Women should not slap their breasts; slap the chest above the breast and around and under the breast only.

3. Use your left palm to slap up and down over your right lung.

4. Use your mind to direct Chi to your chest area.

Slapping is a favorite Taoist technique for eliminating toxins from the skin, muscles, connective tissue, blood vessels and organs. The vibration of the slap beneath the flesh helps to literally shake out impurities and stimulate blood flow. Slapping on bare skin is best but it works through clothes as well—there is just less of a transference of Chi from your hands. It really helps to loosen mucous and clear energy blockages from your lungs.

If you prefer, you can tap on your chest with a loosely held fist, tapping from the wrist and not using the force of the whole forearm. Tapping is just as effective as slapping, it just has a different feel to it. Try them both. They only take fifteen or twenty seconds to perform. Do the tapping whenever you like. Before or after or before and after breathing exercises is a really good time to do them this first week or anytime thereafter.

Regulating the Body: Baduanjin

It is said that Marshall Yueh Fei created eight exercises about eight hundred years ago to keep his soldiers in the field limber and healthy. The exercises were compared to a delicate silk brocade and came to be known as Baduanjin (Pa Tuan Chin) which translates as the Eight Sectioned or Eight Pieces of Brocade. In China today there are many variations of the Eight Pieces of Brocade. There are Standing and Sitting Baduanjin, which are almost totally different from each other. All the standing versions are basically similar with some minor differences in the details of each of the eight exercises. We're going to learn Standing Baduanjin. I will combine the best features of each exercise from the various versions I've learned. I'll also give you some choices so you can do the exercises more or less vigorously.

You can wear soft shoes that are flexible, like sneakers or Chinese Tai Chi shoes. Avoid exercising in hard leather shoes or boots. Take them off and exercise in your socks or barefoot if soft shoes are not available.

The First Piece of Brocade is similar to the Lung Sound Chi Kung.

The First Piece:
Propping Up the Sky with Interlocked Fingers

1. Stand up straight with heels together and feet spread out, duck-style, like the letter V. If you prefer, you can move the feet a few inches apart, but keep them splayed outward duck-style. Your toes should

grip the ground so that the arches of the feet are slightly raised.

2. Your arms should hang naturally at your side. Place the tip of your tongue lightly on the roof of your mouth, just behind your upper teeth.

3. Breathe through your nose. Look straight ahead and relax your joints as best you can.

4. Bring your hands in front of your body, just below the navel, and point the fingers of each hand at each other. Point your palms upward and keep them open. Slowly raise your arms by bending your elbows and bringing your hands, palms facing upward, in front of and close to your body until they reach your upper chest level.

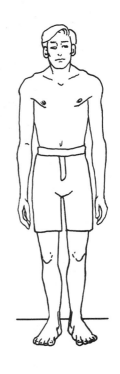

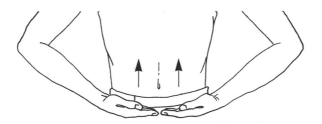

5. At the upper chest level, turn the palms downward and continue turning them outward and upward, until they again face upward, as you continue pushing your hands above your head. When arms are fully raised, interlock your fingers overhead. Palms are turned upward as if you were "propping up the sky." Push upward on the interlocked fingers.

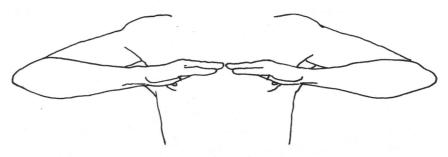

6. Inhale as you raise your arms, simultaneously lift up on your toes, raising your heels off the ground, while continuing to look straight ahead.

7. Exhale as you lower your arms. Disengage your fingers and lower your arms straight outward toward the sides of your body. Slowly sweep the arms down as you exhale. Concentrate on your fingertips

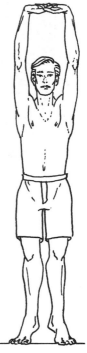

as you slowly lower your arms. Your palms should face outward and finally downward as you lower them.

8. Feel or imagine Chi running to your fingertips, making your hands feel lighter or tingly. Bring your hands back together in front of your body about three inches below your navel as in step 4 above and repeat exercise.

9. Repeat a total of 8 times at each session.

Propping Up the Sky with Interlocked Fingers helps to increase lung capacity, relieve fatigue, improve balance and strengthen the muscles and bones of the back and waist. It also has a general mobilizing effect on the muscles and internal organs of the entire body. In Chinese the full name for this exercise is "Propping Up the Sky With Interlocked Fingers Regulates All the Internal Organs."

In step 2 above, you are instructed to raise the tip of your tongue to the roof of your mouth. This introduces you to one of the most important aspects of the 100 Days of Practice. Raising your tongue to the upper palate connects the Governor and Functional Channels, the body's two main Energy Meridians. One of the primary goals of Taoist training is to connect these two channels. When they are connected and fully opened, so that Chi flows unobstructed through them, this is known as the Microcosmic Orbit. We will work extensively on opening the Microcosmic Orbit later in the training. Raising the tongue to the roof of the mouth was long a Taoist secret. If you don't raise your tongue, the two Channels do not connect. By raising the tongue, the Governor and Functional Channels are connected, even if the Microcosmic Orbit is not yet fully opened. Get into the habit of raising your tongue to the upper palate. For now place the tip of the tongue just behind the upper teeth.

As I mentioned, there are many variations to this exercise. Here are a few:

a. Follow your hands with your eyes as you raise them over your head and as you lower them. It is more difficult to maintain your balance when you look up.

b. Do the exercise with feet shoulder width apart, feet parallel and facing forward, not splayed apart duck-style. Bend the knees slightly. This works the calves differently and makes it more difficult to balance, especially if you look at your hands as you raise and lower them.

c. Don't interlock the fingers. Bring your hands in front of your body in a scooping motion and raise them with fingers pointing toward each other, just an inch or two apart. Do the exercise exactly the same otherwise, but never interlock the fingers.

When hands are fully raised overhead, the palms face upward and the fingers are together and not spread apart and each hand points toward the other with the two middle fingers almost touching. To get the full benefit from this exercise, when hands are raised overhead, push upward toward the ceiling with the thumb, and pull down toward the ground with the pinkie. Don't use too much force. You should feel a stretch in the hand and arm tendons.

d. Do the Healing Sound, S-S-S-S-S-S-S-S as you lower your arms.

e. An easy version—after initially raising the palms overhead and interlocking the fingers, do not lower the arms. Instead keep your hands overhead and as you exhale and lower your heels, relax your arms and turn your palms downward so that they face the top of your head. When you inhale and raise up on your heels, turn the palms upward again. Do this eight times then lower arms out to sides to finish the exercise.

Don't do all these variations at once; first become proficient with the basic exercise Propping Up the Sky With Interlocked Fingers. We will be doing Baduanjin exercises throughout the 100 Days of Practice, so the above variations are more for future reference when you come back to review the instructions. It's still important to keep things simple.

If you can, Propping Up the Sky should be done eight times at least once a day. It is an excellent wake-up exercise. The stretching of the limbs and trunk are similar to the action of stretching and yawning. It gets your Chi flowing.

The Second Piece:
Drawing the Bow on Both Sides

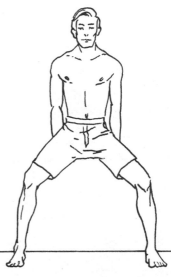

1. Stand up straight with feet parallel, shoulder width apart.

2. Step out to the left with the left foot, so that your feet are greater than shoulder width apart. Your feet remain parallel to each other.

3. Bend both knees and sink down as if you were riding a horse (Horse Stance).

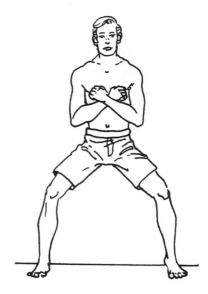

4. Make a fist with both hands and cross hands in front of your chest with left wrist over right wrist.

5. With the left hand, extend the index finger and raise the thumb leaving the middle, ring and pinkie fingers pressed into the palm. Extend your left arm straight out to the left side. The left palm faces away from you so that you are looking at the back of your hand with the index finger pointing up toward the sky, and the thumb pointing in front of you. Keep the other three fingers bent into the outward facing palm.

6. Turn your head to the left with your eyes looking at the raised left index finger as if you were lining up a target.

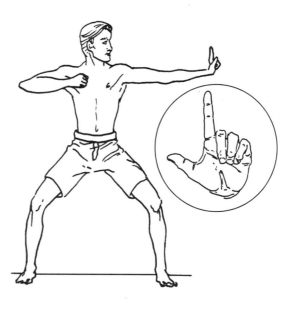

7. At the same time, raise the right fist to shoulder level and pull your right arm, with bent elbow, out to the right side as if you were drawing a bow.

8. Inhale as you extend arms and draw bow. A helpful hint: as you do the exercise, there is a natural tendency to tighten the muscles of the throat; do your best to keep these muscles relaxed. We are generally unaware of the great amount of stress and tension we experience in the throat area.

9. Exhale as you return to the step 4 position with hands crossed in front of your chest, but now with right wrist over left. Repeat exercise to the right side.

10. Repeat at least 4 times to each side, then return to starting position.

Drawing the Bow on Both Sides helps to strengthen the muscles of the neck, chest, shoulders and arms as well as the legs. It also stimulates respiration and blood circulation.

To get more of a stretch, when the arm is extended, pull the raised index finger backward toward your body, keeping the middle, ring and pinkie fingers tucked into the palm. This really works the hand tendons and is good for arthritis sufferers.

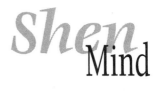

UP TILL NOW, VERY LITTLE has been written about Taoist methods for regulation of Shen, which means both mind and spirit. This is the work that traditionally took 100 days of practice. Unless you are one of the very few who are familiar with Taoist techniques, most of what I will write about over the weeks in the Regulating the Mind section will be totally new to you, even if you are an experienced meditator.

The Taoist techniques of regulating the mind are really what were lost in China when the Taoists were purged. I have met many Chi Kung Masters from China and they, at best, had only rudimentary knowledge of these techniques, especially the more advanced techniques of Internal Alchemy, which we will not deal with in this book. These practices were officially frowned upon by the Communist government. If they exist at all in China today, they do so underground. Most of what I will write about in this section I learned from teachers who were taught by Tao Masters who had fled China to protect their greatest possession. These are authentic teachings that I have structured for a Western audience.

Much of these teachings first appeared in the West around 1930, in a famous and mysterious little book titled *The Secret of the Golden Flower*, translated from an old Chinese manuscript by Richard Wilhelm, with a commentary by Carl Jung, the renowned psychiatrist. In this work, as well as many others, 100 days of concerted effort is the time period set out as necessary to establish a basic foundation in the work. It was the time necessary to bring forth the Golden Flower. Just what this means will be revealed to you as we undertake the 100 Days of Practice.

Initially, we are concerned with calming, quieting and focusing the mind. In Week One I will teach you the first step of the practice known as Sitting and Stilling the Mind. *The Secret of the Golden Flower* calls this the "backward flowing" method. In a few weeks you will understand why.

Sitting and Stilling the Mind: Part One

1. Find a place where no one will disturb you.

2. Sit up straight on a chair with head erect and both feet on the ground. Hold your two hands together in your lap, with the left hand below, palm upward and the right hand above, palm down. (If you already know how to sit comfortably in the Lotus or Semi-Lotus position, then you can do so if you wish. If you don't know it, don't start now, you've got other things to learn and practice.)

3. With eyes open, focus on any point or spot at eye level. The spot can be close or far away, although the recommended distance is 3 to 6 feet, what is more important is that it is directly at eye level. During the course of this first week you can experiment with different distances to judge for yourself what works best for you.

4. Continue to focus on this single spot for at least 3 minutes.

5. For the first 3 days breathe normally. For the next 4 days do deep breathing, but under no circumstance are you to exert yourself as you breathe. If it takes a lot of effort to breathe deeply, don't breathe so deeply.

6. Try to think of nothing except staring at the spot at eye level. Forget your job, any worries and your everyday affairs for just a few minutes.

7. Draw your eyes inward and bring your point of focus to the tip of your nose. To do this, close the eyelids halfway so that it looks like you're squinting, sort of Clint Eastwood style. Look down at the right tip of your nose with your right eye and down at the left tip of your nose with your left eye. Do this for at least 2 minutes.

8. As you look at the tip of your nose be aware of any muscular pull to the left or right. This very often happens because the muscles of one eye are stronger than the other. Try to keep your concentration on the very tip of the nose, which is actually a point you cannot see.

9. Continuing to stare at the tip of your nose, listen to yourself breathing. Try to make your breathing as silent as possible. If you can't hear your breathing at all, this is best. (But this may take many weeks of practice to accomplish. Don't worry if you can still hear your breath despite your best effort to quiet it down.) Continue doing this for at least 3 minutes.

10. If you find that you are getting distracted, then count your breaths to a count of 4. Inhale-2-3-4. Exhale-2-3-4. Inhale-2-3-4. Exhale-2-3-4. Keep your point of concentration on the tip of your nose as you count silently to yourself.

11. Close your eyes, rub your hands together until the palms are hot, and cover your eyes, absorbing the heat from your palms directly into your eyeballs. After about 30 seconds, rub your hands together again, and then massage your face to finish the exercise.

In olden times, Regulating the Mind was referred to as Regulating the Heart. The brain was called the Heavenly Heart. We have now begun the process of Regulating the Heavenly Heart. This is authentic Taoist meditation. Focusing on the tip of the nose is found as the starting point in virtually all authentic Taoist texts. It provides a valuable point of reference for beginning meditators.

One of the problems of beginning meditation is figuring out what to look at or what to think about. The process here is easy: look at the tip of your nose, listen to yourself breathing and think about nothing. It makes it really easy to begin. If you are an advanced meditator, chances are you have not encountered this technique before. Please practice this way. The importance of focusing on the tip of the nose will become more evident in the next couple of weeks. Initially you might feel some eye strain. Bear with it. This is an excellent method for reestablishing the balance in your eye and facial muscles. In a short period of time, it should feel very comfortable. As soon as you focus on the tip of your nose, you will go into a meditative state.

Focusing on the tip of the nose looks funny when performed. At least one text states that when you do it right you "look like a stupid man." That is why it is suggested that you do this exercise in a place where you won't be disturbed. It is a crucial part of the process of Regulating the Mind. Don't avoid it because you think it looks or feels silly. Much of what we will learn in this book will be different, and sometimes startlingly so, from what you have been culturally conditioned to regard as normal or acceptable. That's one of the reasons you're reading this book, isn't it?

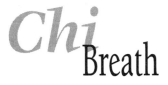

YOU'VE NOW HAD A WEEK to monitor your breath and practice deep breathing. For some of you these exercises were probably pretty easy. For others, conscious breathing may be difficult or laborious.

For those of you experiencing difficulty, the main culprit is usually a tight and stiff diaphragm. If this is your problem, then your diaphragm doesn't move up and down as you inhale and exhale. It feels like a stiff band across the body at the bottom of the rib cage or in the pit of the stomach. Continued breathing practice will, given time, cause your diaphragm to relax and regain its flexibility.

If you're experiencing difficulty with the breathing, keep at it. You might feel some cramping in the diaphragm. Don't worry, this is a good sign. Just like any other muscle, the diaphragm might get sore if it is exercised after a long period (maybe many years) of inactivity. If you're feeling any discomfort, keep doing deep breathing, take a warm bath or massage the diaphragm as you will learn in this week's Self-Massage Rejuvenation section of Regulating the Body.

The diaphragm is a very powerful muscle. It stiffens up in smokers. Tension tightens it. It also tends to stiffen as we age. Shallow breathing doesn't sufficiently exercise the diaphragm and it gets stiff from disuse. A tight diaphragm will result in shallower breathing, and so becomes a vicious circle. The bottom line is that a tight diaphragm will keep you from breathing properly and drawing sufficient oxygen into your system as well as deplete your Vital Energy, leaving you feeling perpetually tired. This is not only unhealthy, but it also blocks the flow of Chi in the middle of your body and strongly contributes to the feeling of aging. A flexible diaphragm will help to restore a feeling of youthfulness and is obviously crucial in making real progress in this work.

This week you will learn the primary Chi Kung breathing technique known as Abdominal Breathing. Abdominal Breathing is nothing more than slightly modified Deep Breathing.

When we do an Abdominal Breath, we inhale, while relaxing and sinking the chest and sternum (breastbone), causing the diaphragm to lower. As it lowers, it puts pressure on the organs below it, especially the adrenal glands which sit on top of the kidneys, and compresses them downward. This provides space for the lower portion of the lungs to fill with air. This downward expansion of the diaphragm, adrenals and kidneys presses down on the abdomen and causes the abdomen to expand outward. When you exhale, the abdomen is contracted inward and pushes up on the organs and diaphragm. Hence the name Abdominal Breathing.

In addition to giving more room for the lungs to breathe and exercising the diaphragm, Abdominal Breathing also gently massages the vital organs and the abdomen. The sinking of the chest and sternum presses on and activates the thymus gland beneath the breastbone, which the Taoists consider to be the most important gland for rejuvenation. As we age, the thymus gland shrinks from the size of a fresh peach to a shriveled-up pit. Activating and restoring the thymus gland is one of the great secret techniques of the Taoists. We begin working on it here.

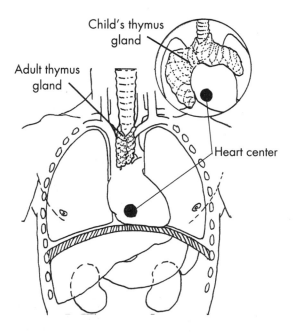

The process of Abdominal Breathing restores to us our original form of breathing. Many Taoist sources refer to it as Natural Breathing because as newborn infants, this is how we breathed. Before birth the infant receives Chi and nourishment from its mother through the umbilical chord, and does not use its lungs to breathe. At birth, the infant starts breathing with its lungs. Initially these lungs are weak. The abdomen assists the lungs in pulling the diaphragm down so that the lower lungs fill with air. Usually we continue to breathe with the help of the abdomen as children. Some of us continue to breathe this way all our lives, but not most of us. All sorts of factors come into play that change our breathing habits and eventually we begin to lose the habit of Abdominal Breathing and do only chest breathing.

The Taoists explain this in terms of Chi pressure. Just as a tire is filled with air creating an internal pressure (pounds per square inch), our body has Chi pressure in our organs and body cavities. At birth and throughout early childhood, our abdomen has more Chi pressure than our lungs. This accounts for an energy-efficient breath in the sense that the lungs don't have to work so hard to bring in air; the Chi pressure in the abdomen does most of the work. However, as we age, if we don't learn how to maintain our internal Chi pressure, we lose this internal pressure and lose the ability to do natural Abdominal Breathing. In other words, our insides get weaker.

Breathing with the lungs, in the chest area only, is energy inefficient. With this type of breathing we rarely fill up more than the upper third of our lungs with air. We use up more energy than we create using the lungs and chest muscles to expand the rib cage as we breathe in, filling only the upper third of our lungs. When we exhale, we seem to collapse inside.

Abdominal Breathing teaches us to increase our internal Chi pressure. With the Chi pressure exerted on the diaphragm and abdomen, the lungs actually expend less energy to completely fill with air. In addition, various internal organs, especially the kidneys, are strengthened by the massaging action of the compression of the expanding diaphragm and abdomen upon inhalation and their subsequent release upon exhalation.

The two kidneys are among the body's most important organs. They serve to filter waste material out of our blood. Our health and longevity depend on them.

The Taoists teach that the kidneys are the storehouses for the body's Original Jing-Essence. This Original Essence is converted into Chi—Life Force Energy—that the body uses to power itself. To conceptualize this, Original Jing is like fuel that is stored in a fuel tank, in this case your kidneys. Chi is that fuel converted into energy. This is what a car's engine does. It converts fuel into energy to power the car. The most important technique for efficient Essence conversion into Chi is Abdominal Breathing. The massaging action of Abdominal Breathing upon the kidneys helps to convert the fuel more efficiently than if you don't do Abdominal Breathing, thus you don't use as much Original Jing. The bottom line—the longer your Original Essence lasts, the longer you live.

As you can see, Abdominal Breathing is vitally important for your health, rejuvenation and longevity. Now let's learn how to do it correctly.

The Abdominal Breath

1. Exhale and pull in the abdomen and stomach toward the spine.

2. Sink and relax the chest and sternum (breastbone). Don't use any force. If you feel a slight pull or flattening of the chest, this is sufficient.

3. Inhale slowly through the nose. Try to keep the chest and stomach flat as you do.

4. Fill the lungs with air. Breathe down to the diaphragm and feel it push downward.

5. The abdomen expands on all sides (not just in front) like a beach ball, as you inhale. There is minimal or no expansion of the chest or stomach region above the navel.

6. When you've reached full capacity without straining yourself, exhale slowly, contracting the abdomen with slight muscular force and relax the diaphragm.

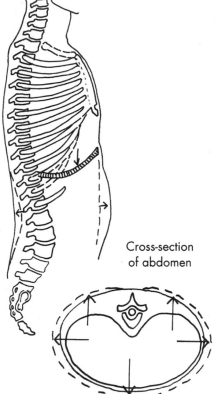

Cross-section of abdomen

7. The inhalation and exhalation should be slow, uninterrupted, of equal length and as silent as you can do them. You have made real progress when the breath becomes imperceptible.

8. Do at least 3 breaths—inhalation and exhalation—initially. If you can, do 9 or more each time you exercise.

The ultimate aim of this exercise is to change your breathing habits so that you restore Abdominal Breathing as your natural way of breathing. This takes time and practice. As you've read above, Abdominal Breathing is really good for you. In many ways it provides the foundation for much of the future work we will be doing during the 100 Days of Practice. Initially you may encounter stiffness, tightness, resistance or soreness. This will pass.

Abdominal Breathing is really easy. Breathe downward and expand the abdomen, exhale and contract the abdomen. Play with the exercise, "Look, Ma, I'm a beach ball." It can be fun if you don't treat it as a chore. Don't forget—you're protecting your greatest possession.

The Second Healing Sound: The Kidney Sound

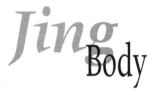

WE'VE ALREADY LEARNED HOW ABDOMINAL Breathing massages the kidneys and gets them to work more efficiently to convert Jing, our Second Treasure, into Chi, our First Treasure, as well as its better known function of removing waste from the blood.

The Healing Sound for the Kidneys is another technique for keeping the kidneys healthy and working efficiently. So let's learn a little more Taoist theory about the kidneys.

In Five Element theory, the kidneys control the Water Element. I am not talking about drinking water here but rather the Force in nature that the Taoists symbolize as Water. Water is pure Yin energy. It is cold energy as compared to its opposite the Fire Element which is pure Yang—hot energy. So the kidneys control the cold Water Element in our bodies.

If we have too much heat in our kidneys, they obviously can't work efficiently to regulate the Water Element and cool off the body. The Healing Sounds work to release heat from the major organs through the fascia. When you release heat from the kidneys they cool off and work better and remain healthier.

Each of the Five Elements is associated with certain negative emotions. We learned the First Week that the negative emotions associated with Metal and the lungs are sadness, grief and depression. The negative emotion associated with Water and the kidneys is fear. Fear is a powerful emotion. Just like the Water Element, it is identified with cold, e.g. "the icy fingers of fear," or "she was frozen with fear." The Kidney Healing Sound will also release excessive cold from the kidneys and neutralize the fear. Neutralizing the negative emotion allows the positive emotion to manifest. For the Water element and the kidneys, the positive emotions are gentleness and wisdom, both of which will break up and overcome fear. Whenever you are frightened, do the Kidney Healing Sound. You'll be surprised at how well it works to dispel the fear.

Excess cold radiating from the kidneys will also weaken the middle and lower back muscles. This is especially true of the Psoas Muscles that surround the spine and run down to either side of the groin and help to keep us erect. The Psoas Muscles hate cold. They freeze up and get stiff if they are not kept warm. The two kidneys are in close proximity to these muscles. Cold kidneys result in cold Psoas Muscles which will get stiff and weak and cut off the free flow of Chi in the Governor Channel going up the back. Later on in the 100 days you'll learn a set of Tao In exercises designed specifically to strengthen the Psoas Muscles. They are among the most important muscles in our body and often among the most difficult to strengthen. The Kidney Healing Sound should help for now.

There are a few versions of the Kidney Healing Sound that I've learned over the years. So I'll use the sound as given in the traditional Taoist literature. It is Chui, pronounced like the two words *chew* (which is pronounced quickly) and *way* (which is pronounced slowly). I'll write it out like this: CH-U-W-A-A-A-Y. When practicing the Healing Sounds, you should begin by doing the Healing Sound for the lungs, S-S-S-S-S-S-S-S, then do the Kidney Sound CH-U-W-A-A-A-Y. So let's do it.

1. Place your awareness on your two kidneys, fist-size organs located on either side of the spine at the bottom of the rib cage on the back. Try to visualize them or feel them or just imagine that they are there.

2. Sit up in a chair with your legs together, ankles and knees touching.

3. Take a deep breath (you can do an Abdominal Breath).

4. As you inhale, bend the trunk of your body forward and hook your hands around your knees, clasping one hand with the other.

5. With hands clasped, pull back on your arms so that you feel a pull on your back where your kidneys are located.

6. Look upward with your eyes and slightly tilt the head back without straining.

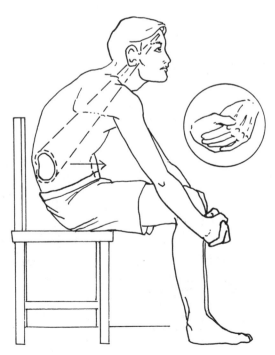

7. Exhale slowly and as silently as you can and make the Healing Sound CH-U-W-A-A-A-Y.

8. As you make the CH-U-W-A-A-A-Y sound, pull in on your stomach area between the bottom of your sternum (breastbone) and your navel. Pull toward the spine and imagine or feel the excess heat or the cold being squeezed out from the fascia surrounding the two kidneys.

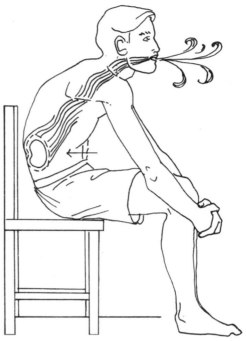

9. Visualize both kidneys bathed in a sapphire blue color and imagine any fear being expelled from the kidneys as you exhale.

10. After finishing exhalation, sit up straight, close your eyes, take a few easy breaths and concentrate on the exchange of energy in the kidney region, before doing another Kidney Healing Sound.

11. Do the CH-U-W-A-A-A-Y sound at least 3 times.

   You should do extra Kidney Sounds in the winter time. Winter is the season associated with the Water Element (autumn is the season of the Metal Element). Each Element had numerous correspondences, an internal organ, a healing sound, a season, negative emotions, positive emotions, color and others which I haven't discussed yet such as external body parts.

Taoist Self-Massage Rejuvenation

The kidneys' main function is to filter waste out of our blood and produce urine. Waste material can collect inside the ducts and tubules of the kidneys in the form of sediment, crystals and uric acid. Hitting the kidneys with the back of the fist helps to shake out any of this harmful material which could impair kidney functioning or form into kidney stones. Hitting the kidneys will also strengthen them and help to relieve back pain. This is an important exercise that should be performed daily.

Hitting the Kidneys

1. Rub your hands together until the palms are hot.

2. Form both hands into fists.

3. The kidneys are on the back side at the bottom of the lowest rib, on both sides of the spine. With the back of each fist, hit around the kidney area.

4. Alternate right fist and then left fist. Hit only as hard as is comfortable from 5 to 10 times on each side.

5. Rub palms together until they are hot and then place them on your back over the two kidneys. Rub your palms up and down, for a few moments, over the kidneys to warm them.

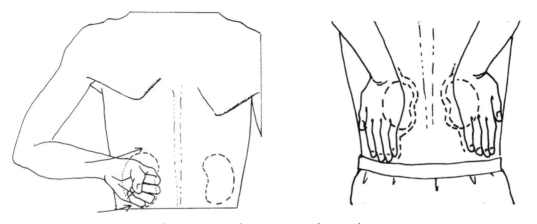

Massaging the Lower Rib Cage and Diaphragm

Chances are you have been feeling tightness, pain or stiffness in the area of the diaphragm at the bottom of the rib cage. This is normal. It happens to most of us. Taoist Self-Massage is used to help relieve any discomfort. Rejuvenation comes by restoring flexibility to the diaphragm.

The diaphragm has a tendency to get tight and stiff and stick to the rib cage. The massage is very simple.

1. Place the back of your index, middle and ring fingers on both hands together, back to back, from the middle knuckle down, so they are pointing at you.

2. Bring the fingers to the bottom of the breastbone in the center of your chest and press into this area with all six fingers.

3. Press in and massage with small circular movements in the solar plexus area at the bottom of the

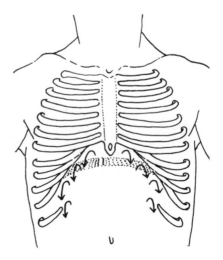

breastbone and then follow the bottom of the rib cage to the left and the right side continuing to massage in small circles. Press inward, then down and around in a clockwise or counter-clockwise direction.

4. From the base of the breastbone, work your way down the rib cage, out to one side of the body, then return to the bottom of the breastbone and massage out to the other side.

5. If you find any particularly sore spots, spend extra time massaging there. Use as much force as you can take.

As you massage, you might feel the stretch of the diaphragm. With just a few sessions of Massaging the Lower Rib Cage and Diaphragm, you will find that breathing should get easier and you can breathe deeper. This is an excellent exercise when you first get up in the morning. It's a good idea to do it before you practice Abdominal Breathing. If you have a lot of pain and stiffness, do it afterwards as well. Work out the soreness; it will disappear if you work at it. It shouldn't take a long time to do. A minute or two on each side is probably enough.

As you become more proficient at Abdominal Breathing, you won't have to massage as often. But it is an area that should be periodically massaged no matter how advanced you become.

Massaging the Ears

According to Taoist theory, the five major internal organs each correspond to an external organ. For the lungs, the external organ is the nose. For the kidneys it is the ears. The Taoists believe there is a connection between the inner and outer organ. The interior organs can be affected by the condition and well-being of the exterior organ.

The ear is a very important organ for maintaining our health and well-being. In addition to its basic function of hearing sounds, the ear has 120 acupuncture points which can affect virtually our entire body. Massaging the ears will not only keep us healthy, but it will also help to prevent hearing loss as we age. There are different exercises for the outer ear and inner ear.

The Outer Ear Massage

The outer ear massage is an extension of the facial massage we learned in Week One. We will continue learning Taoist Self-Massage Rejuvenation for the face and head for the next few weeks.

1. Rub your two hands together until your palms are hot.

2. Bring your left hand up to your left ear and your right hand to your right ear.

Step A—Rubbing the Front and Back of the Ear

3. Keep your hands open with fingers pointed toward the top of your head. Separate the index and middle fingers like a V.

4. Place the index finger behind your ear and the middle finger in front of your ear, so that each ear shell is within the "V" formed by the index and middle fingers.

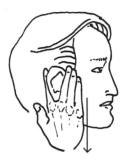

5. Simultaneously rub up and down in front and back of the ears 9 or more times.

Step B—Rubbing the Ear Shells

6. Rub your two hands together again until they get hot.

7. Cover each ear with an open palm with fingers pointed toward the top of your head.

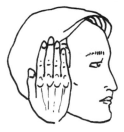

8. Rub each ear shell up and down with the fingers and the palm. This will warm up your entire body and stimulate the autonomic nervous system.

Step C—Stimulating the Ear Lobes

9. Use the thumb and index finger of each hand.

10. Pull down a few times on both ear lobes. Use a little force but not so much that it causes pain.

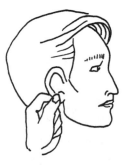

Massaging the Inner Ear: Beating the Heavenly Drum

Because it is inside our head, the inner ear is usually not exercised and weakens as we age, resulting in hearing loss. Since we can't actually touch the inner ear, we use indirect means to reach it. In this exercise we use vibration to strengthen the inner ear. Beating the Heavenly Drum is one of the best known of the Self-Massage Rejuvenation exercises. It is often taught as part of sitting Baduanjin (Eight Pieces of Brocade) which is different from standing Baduanjin.

1. Rub the hands together until hot.

2. Cover your ear shells with your palms.

3. Your fingers point toward the back of the head. Your middle fingers point toward each other and lie on the base of the skull just above the point where the skull ends.

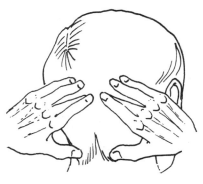

4. Raise the index fingers and place them on top of the middle fingers.

5. Snap the index fingers off the middle fingers so that they tap the base of the skull like a drum. With your palms covering your ears, this might sound quite loud.

6. Repeat 9 or more times.

The flicking of the index finger hitting the base of the skull will cause the bone to vibrate. This will stimulate the inner ear and the nervous system and help us maintain our balance. It should become a lifetime habit and be part of your daily practice.

Baduanjin: The Third and Fourth Pieces

Raising One Hand to Regulate the Spleen and Stomach

1. Stand up straight. You can stand with feet together or feet shoulder width apart, feet parallel, toes facing forward.

2. Both arms and hands hang down naturally on each side of the body.

3. Begin raising the right hand overhead. Turn the right palm to face upward toward the sky. Extend the right arm and raise the right hand over your head with the palm facing upward and your fingers pointing to the left side.

4. Simultaneously press down with the left hand with palm parallel to the ground and fingers of the left hand facing forward.

5. After holding this position for a few seconds, reverse the position of the hands by simultaneously lowering the right hand to the side, palm down and fingers facing forward and raising the left hand overhead, palm facing upward and fingers pointing to the right.

6. Begin inhaling when your rising hand passes your waist level. Exhale as you lower it until you reach your waist level and the opposite hand rises and you begin inhaling again.

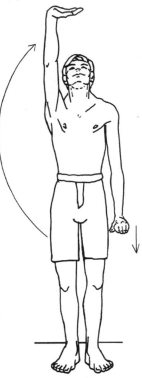

7. Look up toward the raised hand. This provides an excellent stretch for the neck muscles and tendons especially if you turn your head to look upward at the back of your palm.

8. Do each set of alternating left and right hand raising 8 times.

In this third Piece of Brocade, one hand is held up while the other presses down. The vigorous opposite movement of the two hands stretches and stimulates the internal organs and muscles at the same time, especially the liver, gall bladder, spleen, and stomach. This exercise enhances the digestive function, and regular training with it is recommended in the Chinese literature for the prevention and treatment of gastrointestinal diseases.

Turning the Head to Look Back over the Shoulder

1. Stand up straight with feet close together or shoulder width apart as in the previous Piece of Brocade.

2. Arms hang by side of body, hands are open with fingers and palm touching the thigh.

3. Turn your head slowly to the right as far as possible without leaning sideways. Use the eyes to look back over your right shoulder as far to the right as you can.

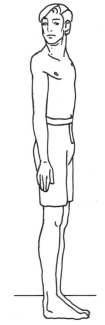

4. Pause for a second or two, then return to starting position.

5. Repeat exercise looking to the left side, then return to starting position.

6. Inhale as you turn your head to look over the shoulder. Exhale as you return to the starting position.

7. Repeat 8 times on each side.

8. For a more strenuous exercise, turn the trunk as well as the head. To do this properly:
   a. Turn the trunk to the right using the muscles at the waist.
   b. Next, turn the muscles in the middle of the back, all the way to the right.
   c. Next, turn the right shoulder as far to the right as possible.
   d. Now turn the head and look over the right shoulder.
   e. Return to starting position and
   f. Repeat on the left side.

The Fourth Piece of Brocade aids in strengthening the muscles surrounding the eye sockets and increases mobility of the eyes. It strengthens the neck muscles and prevents ailments and injuries to the cervical vertebra in the neck. It stimulates blood circulation to the head and brain and improves the balancing function while eliminating tiredness, dizziness and other disturbances to the central nervous system. It is especially recommended for sufferers of hypertension and arteriosclerosis.

Sitting and Stilling the Mind: Part Two

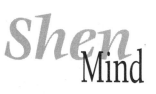

IN WEEK ONE WE BEGAN the method of Sitting and Stilling the Mind. I hope you have continued the practice. It is most important to learn to focus the mind in order to overcome distraction. We learned to sit and focus the eyes on some point in front of us at eye level and then after a few minutes bring our focus to the tip of our nose while half closing the eyelids. While we are doing this, we are supposed to clear our minds and think of nothing and listen to ourselves breathing.

While it is easy for me to tell you to think of nothing, in actuality this is most difficult to achieve. Thoughts whiz through the mind. They seem to arise out of nowhere. If we consciously try to stop them, we quickly realize that they are beyond our conscious control. The Taoists have long understood that you cannot overcome consciousness by using consciousness. In other words you cannot use thoughts and the thinking process to turn off thoughts and the thinking process. The correct approach is indirect.

In Week Two we will continue the process begun in Week One called Sitting and Stilling the Mind using the Backward Flowing Method. From the tip of the nose, we will bring our focus up the nose to the "little bump" about one-half inch from the bridge of the nose. After a minute or so here, we will bring the focus up all the way to the point between the two eyes—the Yin Tang—which we learned to massage in Week One, and fix our consciousness there. This is the beginning of true meditation. With practice, the thought process will start to slow down. You will be able to observe your thinking process. By observing your thoughts you will be able to trace where they arose in your mind, where thoughts begin and where thoughts fade out and disappear. This is the best we can do. When we learn to trace thoughts back to their place of origin they tend to quiet down and then ultimately stop of their own volition. But this won't happen by itself—you must do the practice.

1. Begin as in Week One by taking a seated position on a chair holding your palms in your lap, left palm up covered by the right palm down.

2. With eyes open, focus on a spot at eye level for 1 or 2 minutes.

3. Draw your eyes inward and bring your point of concentration to the tip of your nose with your eyelids closed halfway. Do this for 2 or 3 minutes while you listen to yourself do Abdominal Breathing as quietly as you can. (If Abdominal Breathing is initially too distracting, just try to breathe as silently as you can.)

4. Raise your point of focus from the tip of your nose to a point two-thirds the way up the nose, where many of us have a small (or not so small) bump about one half-inch from the bridge (top) of the nose. Keep the eyelids half-closed. Continue concentrating on this point for one or two minutes while you continue to listen to yourself breathing as silently as you can.

5. Bring your point of concentration to the point between the two eyes, the Yin Tang. Your eyelids may squint a little more, but don't allow them to close. It is more as if you are focusing your thoughts on this spot, which is also known as the Third Eye Point, than actually seeing it. If you could see yourself, it would appear as if you are crossing your eyes.

6. Continue breathing silently.

7. Listen to any thought in your head. If there are many thoughts, just pick one at a time and listen to it. Try to seek out where in your mind the thought arose. You might find that it appeared spontaneously out

of a particular spot in your brain, or from behind your eyes or the back of your head. You will find that certain thoughts always seem to arise from the same place in your mind. Do this for 3 minutes or more. If you find yourself getting distracted or lost in your thoughts, focus back on the tip of your nose, then bring your point of concentration to the "bump" one half-inch below the bridge and then after a few seconds back to the Third Eye point.

8. You can count your breaths to a count of 4 to maintain or restore concentration at any time during the exercise.

9. Close your eyes, rub your hands together until the palms are hot, and cover your eyes, absorbing the heat from your palms directly into your eyeballs. After about 30 seconds, rub your hands together again, then massage your face, nose and ears to finish the exercise.

There is a lot of new material here. You might prefer to work on the "bump" point, two thirds of the way up the nose, for a few days before moving up to the Third Eye point. It is important for you to work at your own pace. If you need more time at a certain set of exercises, take it. It is all right to go slowly. If it takes you fifteen or sixteen or twenty-six weeks to complete this practice, that's all right too. Just don't slow down so much that you stop altogether. If you want to move ahead more rapidly, it's fine to read ahead and practice the Second Treasure—Regulating the Body—exercises including Self-Massage Rejuvenation, Six Healing Sounds and the moving exercises. As far as the First Treasure—Regulating the Breath—exercises, you probably can read and practice a week or two ahead but I would advise against any more than that. If you try to do too much too soon, you will not establish a firm foundation in the breathing practice. As far as the Third Treasure—Regulating the Mind—exercises are concerned, don't move ahead more rapidly then set out here. It is important to move slowly with the Third Treasure exercises so that each step is mastered before you move onto the next.

Continue Abdominal Breathing as you learned it in Week Two. If you can, expand the time you practice to between five and ten minutes a day. You can do it pretty much anywhere and any time, when you first get up, while taking a shower, while commuting to 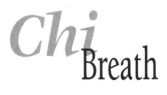 work, while walking, while sitting at your desk, while doing the Regulating the Mind exercises. The only time not recommended to practice is within one hour of eating a meal and even longer after a heavy meal.

Abdominal Breathing takes a lot of practice before it becomes habitual. So please remember to do it every day. It does get easier with practice. If you find you are still feeling discomfort, do as much as you can and continue to Massage the Diaphragm as you learned last week.

This is an important week as we continue on our 100 Days of Practice. We will learn the Healing Sound for the Liver, Taoist Self-Massage Rejuvenation for the 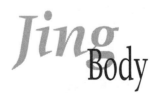 eyes, the fifth and sixth Pieces of Brocade and we will begin learning the sexual techniques.

The Third Healing Sound: The Liver Sound

The liver is the largest gland in the body. It weighs three pounds, more or less, and is found on the right side of the upper abdomen at the bottom of the rib cage. It is a soft, elastic organ that is kept in place by ligaments attached to the diaphragm, abdominal wall, stomach and intestines. The liver has more than 500 separate functions. It produces bile which controls the breakdown, digestion and excretion of fats from our body. It converts protein and fat into carbohydrates and stores these carbohydrates. It regulates our blood sugar level. It acts to detoxify our body of drugs and alcohol. It also acts as a storehouse of vitamins, minerals, metals and a host of other necessary body substances. In a way it is the body's pharmacy, storing and dispensing medicines and vitamins.

A healthy liver is vital to the body's health and longevity. The Taoists developed many techniques and exercises to accomplish these ends. To the Taoists the liver is the manifestation and the storehouse of the Wood Element in the body. The Wood Element has a generating quality, symbolized by wood growing out of the earth. The Wood Element is also stored in the gall bladder which is attached to the underside of the liver and is the storehouse of the bile produced by the liver. Wood energy is warm and moist. It acts together with the Metal energy of the lungs, which is cool and dry, to regulate body temperature from extremes of hot and cold.

The negative emotion associated with the liver is anger. Too much anger causes the liver to overheat and harden. In some people it feels like a big, hard piece of wood, underneath and below the right rib cage. The Liver Healing Sound aids in releasing the excess heat from the liver. Releasing this heat reduces and dissolves anger. Anger is a very unhealthy emotion, which often leads to explosive or self-destructive behavior. It creates rifts between and separates people from one another. Too much heat in the liver causes anger. So we will now learn how to do the Liver Healing Sound and begin the process of changing the negative emotion of anger into the liver's positive emotion which is kindness.

The eyes are the external organs associated with the liver. In Taoist terms, the eyes are considered the external openings for the liver. The eyes are vitally important to the process of Chi Kung. Many of the exercises in this Third Week involve the eyes. I will speak about them at greater length in the next section on Self-Massage Rejuvenation.

In many ways the transformation of negative emotions into their positive counterparts is the most important part of this training. It is also among the most difficult aspects to write about. This transformation results in what the Taoists called the creation of Virtuous Energy. This is the long-time secret side effect of the practice; as you learn it and do it you become a better person or what the I Ching refers to as the Superior Man (or Woman). Not in any egotistical sense, but rather you become a more moral, virtuous person, better able to cope with and deal with the world around you.

1. Sit up in your chair and place your awareness on your liver.

2. Let your arms hang at your sides and turn your hands so that your palms face outward.

3. Take a long deep breath as you slowly raise your arms out to your sides, palm upward. Continue raising your arms until they are overhead.

4. Look up and follow the movement of your arms above your head with your eyes.

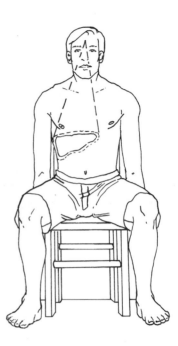

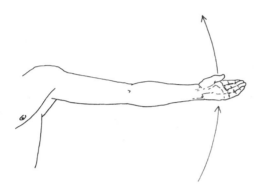

5. Interlock the fingers of both hands overhead. Your palms now face down toward the top of your head.

6. Rotate your palms so they face upward, toward the ceiling.

7. Push up on the heel of both palms and bend from the waist a little bit to the left so that there is more of a stretch on the right side, which is the liver side.

8. Open your eyes wide as you exhale and sub-vocally make the Liver Healing Sound: SH-H-H-H-H-H-H.

9. Visualize and feel that your liver is enclosed in a sac and that excess heat is being expelled through the fascia sac.

10. Visualize your liver bathed in emerald green light and as you exhale, anger is expelled from your liver, right through your skin, like gray smoke.

11. When you have fully exhaled, separate your fingers and slowly lower your hands and arms out to your sides and continue moving them

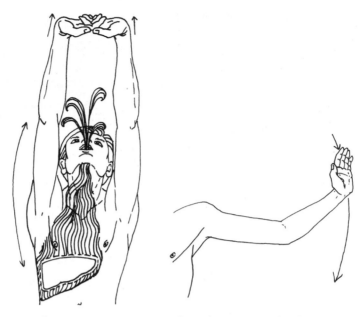

down to the starting position. When done properly, the arms seem to float outward and downward.

12. Rest for a few moments, breathing normally with your mind focused on your liver.

13. Do the Liver Healing Sound SH-H-H-H-H-H-H-H at least 3 times a day.

For your daily practice, you should do all three Healing Sounds for the lungs, kidneys and liver. The Healing Sounds themselves have a healing effect of their own, even if you don't do the Chi Kung movements.

Taoist Self-Massage Rejuvenation: The Eyes

In Taoist theory, the two eyes are Yang and the rest of the body is Yin. The eyes are considered to be the positive poles of the body. They have the power and potential to transform the negative-Yin energy inside of us into positive-Yang energy. They are used to guide the flow of Chi throughout our body and to heal ourselves of latent ailments.

In our modern world much stress is placed upon the eyes as we engage in activities such as driving, watching television, working with computers and reading. Since the eyes are directly connected to our nervous system, stress on our eyes creates stress on our nervous system. Generally we are not consciously aware of this happening.

Weeks One and Two of the Regulating the Mind exercises involved using the eyes to focus first on the tip of the nose, then on the bump of the nose and finally on the bridge of the nose between the two eyes. In doing these exercises, you might have experienced some strain in the eye muscles. The exercises in this section will help to relieve pain and tension in and behind the eyes, strengthen the eyes and eye muscles and reduce wrinkles around the eyes. You will probably find that there is a tremendous amount of tension and pain in your eyes and eye muscles that you were not aware of. All this stress and pain affects your entire nervous system and body as well as your ability to do the Third Treasure—Regulating the Mind exercises.

As already mentioned, in Taoist theory the eyes are linked to and are the external openings of the liver. Healthy eyes help to maintain and are a sign of a healthy liver. In addition, different parts of the eyes are linked to all five of the major Yin internal organs. The whites of the eyes are linked to the lungs, the pupils are linked to the kidneys, the irises are linked to the liver, the corners of the eyes to the heart and the lids of the eyes to the spleen. We will begin working with these five parts of the eyes in this week's Regulating the Mind section when we take the first step of Smiling into our Eyes.

Massaging the Eyeballs and Sockets

1. Rub your hands together until they are hot.

2. Close your eyes.

3. Take a deep breath and hold it while using your mind to mentally direct Chi to both your eyes.

4. Use your middle fingertip to massage the center of both your eyeballs through your closed eyelids. Massage gently 6 to 9 times clockwise then the same number counterclockwise.

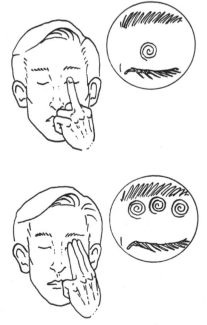

5. Exhale and take another deep breath directing Chi to both eyes.

6. Use the index, middle and ring fingers of both hands to massage the upper portion of the eye, placing the fingertips just below the eye sockets. Massage 6 to 9 times clockwise and counterclockwise.

7. Repeat step 6 for the lower part of the eyes around the bottom socket of the eyes.

8. Make a fist with both hands and rub the sides of the bent index fingers together until hot.

9. Use the side of each index finger to massage the eye sockets. Press as deep into the space between the eyeball and the bone of the eye socket as you can take. Use the knuckle of each index finger to press into the inner corner of each eye, then press the sides of each index finger around the edge of the eye socket, moving toward the outer corner of the eyes. Do this 6 to 9 times for upper and lower sockets.

Be especially aware of painful spots. These points must be massaged until the pain disappears. This will probably take a number of sessions. If you stop massaging the eyes regularly, the pain will probably return. If you wear eyeglasses or spend many hours a day staring at something straight ahead of you like a television or computer screen, you might find your eye muscles have become somewhat rigid. When you first begin massaging, these muscles might feel numb. After a little massaging, the blood and Chi flow will increase to these muscles and you might then experience intense pain. Daily massage will help to restore flexibility and relieve the pain. You may often find that as you start massaging your eyes, muscles in the neck, shoulders and underarms might spontaneously relax. Most of us have an unbelievable amount of stress and tension locked up behind our eyes.

Pulling in the Eyeballs

Pulling in the eyeballs is one of the best exercises for the eye muscles. It also exercises the brain, senses, glands and internal organs. We generally do not exercise our eye muscles and as a result they tend to weaken as we age. This is a very simple exercise to help restore the eye muscles' natural muscle tone.

1. Rub your palms together until hot then cup both eyes with the palms.

2. Inhale and relax.

3. Exhale and tighten and contract your anus and pull up on your sexual organs.

4. Pull in on your eyeballs so that it feels as if they are being pulled back into your eye sockets.

5. Inhale and relax.

6. Repeat 3 to 6 times per session.

   This exercise introduces us to one of the most important concepts in the entire practice of Chi Kung: Perineum Power.

The perineum is part of the Pubococcygeus or PC Muscle that runs from above the sexual organs to the coccyx (tailbone). The perineum itself is located between the back of the sexual organs and the front of the anus. It is the lowest point on the torso of our body. This point is known as the Hui-yin, which in Chi Kung training often refers to not only the perineum, but the anus and the sexual organs and surrounding muscles, as well. Hui-yin means collection point of the Yin energy and is also called the Gate of Life and Death. It is divided into various parts that we will explore as we continue with our 100 Days of Practice.

For now, we should be aware of the three distinct parts of the Hui-yin. There is the perineum itself, which is at the bottom of all the body's internal organs. It must withstand the combined weight and pressure of these organs and hold them in place. When the perineum is weak, the internal organs sag down and lose energy.

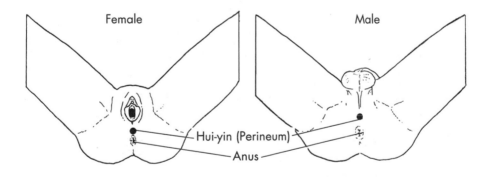

The perineum lies between the body's two main energy gates. There is the Front Gate or sexual organs. From here we can easily lose Jing from ejaculation or menstruation. We also lose Chi if the muscles of the sexual organs are weak and fail to seal off the opening of the penis or vagina.

The Second Gate is the anus. We leak energy from the anus if it is not sealed or closed tight. When it is sealed, it is like tying a knot in a balloon to keep the air from escaping; it keeps our Chi from escaping. It can also be used to direct Chi to various points of the body.

At this stage in your practice it is sufficient to contract and pull up the entire PC Muscle, including anus and sexual organs, as you pull in on your eyeballs. You should sense some connection between the eyes and the Hui-yin. You can feel a stronger pull in the eyes above when you use Perineum Power down below. There will be more about this subject later in the chapter.

Getting the Tear Out and Growing the Positive Energy

So many of the Self-Message Rejuvenation exercises seem to be so basic that they appear to be childlike in their simplicity. This is just such an exercise. It is one of the most startling and effective exercises I have ever learned. Over the years, I've learned many variations of this exercise, some simple, some much more complicated. But I promised to keep things simple so I'll give you the basic exercise with a few suggested variations at the end.

The premise is easy: we stare at some point while keeping our eyes open without blinking. Within a short time, the eyes will begin to tear. This is the desired result. These tears are not the same kind of tear you shed when you are crying. The Taoists believe that toxins burn out of the body through the eyes. These tears will be salty and may have an unpleasant smell because they are the residue of internal combustion. Getting the Tear Out causes the positive-Yang energy of the eyes to increase. As mentioned, the entire body is negative-Yin and only the eyes are positive-Yang. This positive-Yang Energy is used to rid the body of toxins and ailments. If the exercise is done regularly over a period of time, its curative and rejuvenating effects are truly remarkable.

1. Hold one index finger straight up about 8 inches in front of your eyes.

2. Take a deep breath and open your eyes wide and stare at your fingertip without blinking.

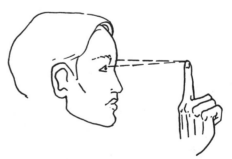

3. Hold your breath for a few seconds before exhaling slowly. Continue with deep abdominal breaths and holding the breath before each exhalation.

4. You will soon feel a burning sensation in the eyes. Do your best not to give in to the temptation to close your eyes until you feel a tear gather or fall in both eyes.

5. Rub your palms together until hot. Close your eyes and cover them with your palms. Absorb the warmth (Chi) from your palms into your eyeballs.

6. Circle your closed eyes completely around the eye sockets at least 3 times clockwise (from the top of the eye come down on the left side and up on the right) and an equal number counterclockwise. This is an important part of the practice and can be performed independently, at any time, to exercise the eyes.

As variations, you can:
a. Stare at a dot on a wall 5 to 6 feet in front of your eyes.
b. Stare at the blue part of the flame of a lighted candle.
c. Stare into your eyes in a mirror.

As you become more proficient at keeping your eyes open, you can increase the length of time you stare without blinking to 15 minutes or more. This exercise should be performed every day this week. Thereafter it is recommended that you do it at least a few times weekly. This is a wonderful, simple exercise, but it is often difficult to motivate yourself to do it because it can be a little uncomfortable. It is a truly beneficial exercise that should not be ignored.

Sexual Kung Fu

Regulation of the Body concerns the Taoist's Second Treasure: Jing. Jing is our Essence and the most powerful form of Essence is Sexual Energy. In this early stage of our training, we are concerned with building up our strength and stamina and learning new ways to get in touch with our bodies.

Jing-Essence is converted inside the body into Chi-Energy. If more Jing is available to us this means that there is more Essence available for conversion into Energy. Thus a primary goal of the Regulating the Body exercises is to increase the body's reservoir of Jing.

The easiest way to increase Essence is through stimulation. Our first steps in Seminal and Ovarian Kung Fu are designed to increase our production of sexual energy. For men this involves massaging the testicles and for women massaging the breasts to stimulate the ovaries.

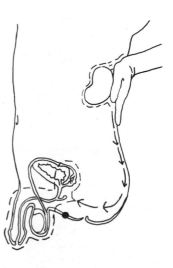

Seminal Kung Fu for Men: Part One

1. Rub your palms together until they are hot then place them on your back over your kidneys. Rub your palms over your kidneys for 15 to 30 seconds to warm them.

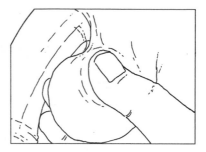

2. Breathe deeply and feel or imagine energy descending from the kidneys, down your back to the sexual organs.

3. Rub your palms together again and gently massage each testicle for about a minute. Massage each testicle between the tip of your thumb on one side, and your index, middle and ring fingertips on the other side. Do not use any force or pressure.

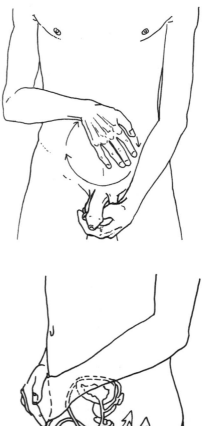

4. Cup your testicles in your left hand. Place your right palm over your navel and circle your hand around the navel 36 times in a clockwise (from above down on the left side then up on the right side) direction. Circle and massage the lower abdomen as you do this.

5. Reverse hands and hold testicles in your right hand as you circle the navel and massage the lower abdomen 24 times in a counterclockwise direction.

6. Place the left palm on your lower abdomen just above your penis and place your right palm on top of your left. The two hands are covering an important energy center known as the Sperm Palace.

7. Pull in on the muscles around your eyes and use perineum power. Feel a light contraction and stimulation in your perineum, the tip of your penis, the urogenital diaphragm inside the penis and the anal sphincter.

8. Pause and feel the Jing expand in the Sperm Palace at the base of the penis, where the organ joins the body and the surrounding area.

9. Use your mind and look down with your eyes to guide the Essence from the Sperm Palace, down your legs and into the ground. If you

feel nothing, just use your imagination. The Essence might feel thick and heavy as it splits in two and runs down through your thighs, through your knees, down your calves and into your ankles. It spreads out through your feet and into your toes and exits your body and descends into the earth from the center of the soles of your feet.

10. Use your imagination to visualize the Jing spreading out and descending into the Earth like the roots of a tree. (If you practice in a high-rise building, imagine the Jing spreads out into the floor beneath your feet.)

Jing-Essence in the form of Sexual Energy feels much heavier than Chi. Its tendency is to sink downward. Thus, it should be fairly easy for you to feel or imagine the Essence moving down your legs and into the ground. It is much more difficult to get the Jing Chi to rise upward.

In this exercise we are actually learning to move the Jing Chi in both directions. By feeling the connection between the eyes and the perineum as we pull on them, we are laying the foundation for later exercises where we will actually learn how to raise the Sexual Energy up the spine.

By lowering the Essence down our legs and into the ground, we are also beginning to learn how to "root" ourselves to the earth. This is an important concept to the practice. When we are rooted to the earth, we are protecting ourselves from getting too "spacey" or detached from the earth. In Chi Kung practice we seek to be firmly rooted in the everyday world: we don't do it to avoid or escape our responsibilities in "the real world." Rooting practice, in time, will also provide a source of strength as we become more proficient. The earth itself will support us and allow us to draw power from the ground beneath us. Many of the Taoist practices are very literal in the sense that their names are a description of the practice. A Taoist absolutely believes that he or she can move the Essence and Energy in their body or out of their body. It is not even questioned. In China you would have been brought up believing in it as part of the natural scheme of things. In the West these concepts are practically unknown. But again there is nothing Chinese about your Essence or your Life Force Energy; everyone has them, whatever their race or gender. They were discovered in China and it has just taken a long time for these ideas to reach the West. There are many practitioners of Chi Kung in China who predict that Chi Kung will become a major force for health prevention and maintenance around the world in the twenty-first century.

You can do this exercise when you shower or any time during the day when you're alone and won't be interrupted. It is not a good exercise to do before you go to sleep because you will build up energy that can keep you awake. You also don't want to become too sexually aroused so that all the Jing Chi is lost through intercourse or masturbation. The idea here is to build up the Sexual Energy and feel it connect with the eyes, spread out into the abdomen and down the legs and into the ground. Remember we want to conserve as much sperm as possible, not lose as much as possible.

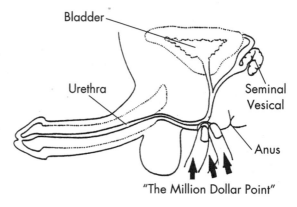

Bladder

Urethra

Seminal Vesical

Anus

"The Million Dollar Point"

If you feel yourself getting too aroused, stop and do some rapid Abdominal Breathing and look up and to the left with your eyes. Use the index, middle and ring fingers of either hand to locate the depression in the perineum behind the testicles, but closer to the anus, and press inward and upward with the middle finger. The Taoists refer to this as the Million Dollar Point. You'll have to feel around for it before you do the exercise. Just pressing on the perineum will not stop the flow of sperm. You must find the small depression, your Million Dollar Point. By experimentation, you should be able to locate it. By practicing using masturbation, you can learn to have an orgasm but prevent the loss of sperm. Afterward, massage the perineum with the three fingers. You should have fun learning. The Taoists had nothing against having fun.

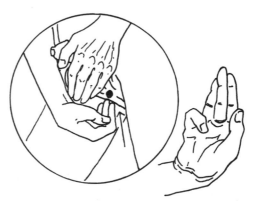

Ovarian Kung Fu for Women: Part One

1. Rub you hands together until they are hot.

2. Cover each breast with a palm and begin to circle and massage. Circle by bringing the two hands close together from below the breasts upward toward the center of the chest then over the top of the breasts and finally outward and downward. Do this 9 to 18 times.

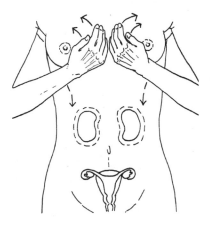

3. Reverse direction and massage from above breast, downward toward middle of the chest then below and massage upward toward the outside of the breast.

4. Rest with fingertips lightly touching the nipples.

5. Feel the Jing descend downward and backward toward your two kidneys. You might experience this as a sexual feeling or as warmth.

6. Place your palms on your lower back over the two kidneys and massage this area for 15 to 30 seconds.

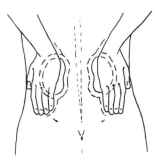

7. Put your mind on your Ovarian Palace, which includes the area of the vagina and the two ovaries on either side of and slightly above the vagina. Feel the Jing descend from the kidneys down into the Ovarian Palace.

8. Move your palms down and cover the Ovarian Palace.

9. Pull in on the eye muscles and use perineum power by closing and tightening the lips of the vagina and pulling upward while simultaneously tightening and pulling up on the anus.

10. Pause and feel the energy expand in the sexual area.

11. Use your mind and look down with your eyes to guide the Essence from the Ovarian Palace, down your legs and into the ground. If you

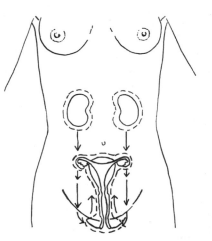

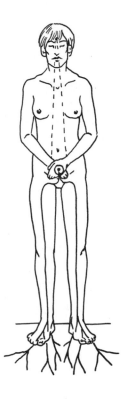

feel nothing, just use your imagination. The
Essence might feel thick and heavy as it splits
in two and runs down through your thighs,
through your knees, down your calves and into
your ankles. It spreads out through your feet
and into your toes and exits your body and
descends into the earth from the center of the
soles of your feet.

12. Use your imagination to visualize the Jing spreading out and descending into the Earth like the roots of a tree.

This exercise can be done in the shower or any time you have privacy.
It can be done at night but be aware of the potential for it arousing you
sexually. If this should occur, it is permissible to relieve the sexual
arousal by intercourse or masturbation. Women do not lose Jing through
sexual activity.

The comments after the description of the Seminal Kung Fu Part One
exercise regarding rooting and raising Jing apply equally to women.

Badjuanjin: The Fifth and Sixth Pieces

The Fifth Piece:
Swinging the Head and Buttocks to Extinguish Fire in the Heart

1. Stand with feet facing forward about three feet apart.

2. Bend both knees and sink down as if you were riding a horse.

3. Place your palms on your thighs with fingers on the inner part of the
thighs and the thumb on the outer part pointing backwards.

4. Lower the head and bend the trunk of your body forward.

5. Swing the head and trunk to the left side while you simultaneously swing the buttocks in the opposite direction to the right. Stretch the right leg to aid the movement. Inhale as you swing the head and buttocks.

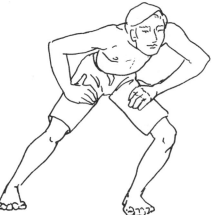

6. Return to the forward position as you exhale.

7. Repeat the exercise by swinging head and trunk to the right side and buttocks to the left as you stretch the left leg and inhale.

8. Return to forward position as you exhale.

9. Repeat a total of 8 times in each direction.

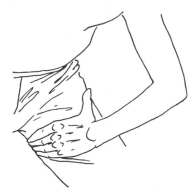

This exercise aids in "extinguishing fire in the heart," a traditional Chinese medical term which means overcoming strain in the nervous system caused by stress and physical exertion which is not eased through rest.

The Sixth Piece:
Grasping the Toes with Both Hands to Reinforce the Kidneys

1. Stand up straight with feet pointed forward no more than one foot apart (it can be less). Arms are at your sides.

2. Place the back of both hands against your lower back and bend your upper body backward and look up toward the ceiling with your eyes. Pause for a moment.

3. Bend slowly forward from the waist, keeping both legs straight and not bending the knees. Exhale as you bend forward.

4. Continue bending forward until you can reach down

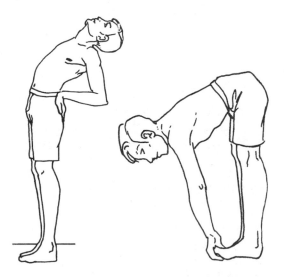

with both hands and grasp and pull up the toes on both feet. If you cannot reach the toes, try to touch your ankles with your fingertips.

5. Return to starting position as you inhale.

6. Repeat a total of 8 times.

In this exercise the muscles of the waist and back are stretched and contracted helping to prevent and cure strains. It also works to improve the functioning of the kidneys and the adrenal glands. If you suffer from hypertension or arteriosclerosis, it is recommended that you do not bend your head too far forward when doing this exercise.

Smiling into the Eyes

Shen Mind

THIS WEEK WE CONTINUE THE process of Sitting and Stilling the Mind by adding the technique of Smiling into the Eyes.

We've already discussed the importance of the eyes in Chi Kung practice. This exercise aids in relieving stress and tension in and around the eyes, and also helps in the ability to direct the flow of Chi.

Last week we began observing our thoughts and trying to trace thoughts back to their place of origin. You might have become aware that many thoughts seem to arise spontaneously in and around the eye region. The Taoists long ago realized that many of the random thoughts that clutter our head are the result of tension or pain in our head and body. This is especially true of the eyes. As you've learned this week, we often suffer from chronic stress and pain in and around the eyes that we're often not even aware of. The constant "nagging" effect of this stress and pain results in our mind misinterpreting the message and verbalizing it. For instance, a muscle behind the eyes becomes tight and painful. It sends out this message to the pain receptors in the brain. This message is nonverbal. However, the brain interprets it as pain. As the condition becomes chronic, the message of pain is constantly being sent out. In time the brain begins to interpret the message as "I'm in pain" or "I hurt, I hurt." The message is repeated over and over, endlessly. This is happening on a level that your conscious mind is not aware of. In this manner, messages of pain and stress are verbalized in the mind and begin to take on a life of their own. Since we are not consciously aware of what's happening, these messages proliferate over time to fill our head with endless chatter that seems to be spontaneously generated in our head for no apparent reason. Most of it is simply pain and stress, verbalized by our brain in a futile effort to interpret the message.

As the stress and pain in and around the eyes is reduced, you will find that the constant chatter is also reduced and it will become easier for you to observe this reduced flow of thoughts and trace them back to their place of origin. Along with massage and getting a tear out as taught in Week Three, Smiling into the Eyes is a most important technique and lays the foundation for the technique called the Inner Smile which we will continue working with over the next few weeks.

1. Do the practice of Sitting and Stilling the Mind as taught in Week Two. First, briefly focus on a point in front of you. Next squint your eyes and focus on the tip of your nose for a minute or two, then raise your point of focus two-thirds of the way up your nose to the little bump for a minute or two. Next move your point of focus and concentration to the spot between the two eyes, the Third Eye Point, and let it remain there for a minute or two.

2. Close your eyes.

3. Use your imagination or visualizing powers to envision the Sun if it's during the daytime, or the Moon if it is nighttime, directly in front of your eyes. This Sun or Moon has a smiling face and the face is smiling directly into your eyes. You can also visualize the smiling face of a loved one if you find this easier.

4. Direct the incoming smiling energy from the Sun, Moon or loved one into the outer corner of your left eye. Feel the outer corner of your left eye begin to relax and smile.

5. Lift up the left corner of your mouth into a smile. Feel the connection between the smiling left corner of your mouth and the smiling outer corner of your left eye. Feel the left side of your face seem to rise up and relax.

6. Repeat this procedure for the outer corner of your right eye and the right corner of your mouth.

7. Smile into the inner corner of the left eye.

8. Repeat for the inner corner of the right eye.

9. Draw smiling energy from the Sun or Moon into the left pupil (the black central part) and feel the pupil fill with smiling energy.

10. Repeat for the right pupil and feel the right pupil fill with smiling energy.

11. Draw smiling energy into the left iris (the circular colored part of the eye surrounding the pupil) and feel the left iris fill with smiling energy. Inhale an Abdominal Breath then exhale and pull in on the circular muscle of the iris and pull up on the anus to help you feel and activate the iris. Inhale and release.

12. Repeat for the right iris and exhale and pull in on the right iris and pull up on the anus. Inhale and release.

13. Smile into the entire white part of the left eye, on the inside of the eye as well as the outside and feel the eyeball fill with smiling energy.

14. Repeat for the white of the right eye and the inside of the eye.

15. Smile into the upper left eyelid and feel it fill with smiling energy.

16. Smile into the upper right eyelid and feel it fill with smiling energy.

17. Smile into the lower left eyelid and feel it fill with smiling energy.

18. Smile into the lower right eyelid and feel it fill with smiling energy.

19. Keep your eyes closed and put your awareness onto the tip of your nose. Bring your awareness up to the bump on your nose and then to the Third Eye.

20. Smile into your Third Eye. Draw the smiling energy of the Sun if it's daytime, or the Moon if it's nighttime, or the smiling face of a loved one into your Third Eye area. Feel this area relax as it fills with smiling energy.

21. Draw the smiling energy into your head. Imagine that you are using a line of sight that begins at the tip of your nose, traveling up your nose, past the bump to the Third Eye and continue backward about 3 inches into your brain. Remain here for a few minutes. Observe your thoughts or just sit quietly.

22. Rub your hands together until hot then massage your face and cover your eyes with your palms and absorb the heat for a few seconds before opening your eyes.

week four

Abdominal Breathing and Perineum Power: Part One

I HOPE THAT AS WE begin this fourth week that you have been doing the Abdominal Breathing exercises daily. This week we will combine Abdominal Breathing with Perineum Power, which we began working with last week. With this type of breathing we are laying the foundation for many of the exercises we will be doing in future weeks.

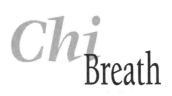

The method is easy. You pull up on the perineum and anus only. Do not pull up on the sexual organs in this exercise. As you progress with this work, you will find that you can differentiate between different parts of the perineum area such as front, back and sides. For now you are just getting familiar with working with this area, so try to pull up only on the perineum muscle between the sexual organs and the anus itself. In this exercise you pull up only on exhalation and not on inhalation. Here is a full description of the Abdominal Breath with Perineum power:

1. Exhale and pull in the abdomen and stomach toward the spine.

2. The chest and sternum (breastbone) relax and sink. Don't use any force. You should feel a slight pull or flattening of the chest.

3. Inhale slowly through the nose. Try to keep the chest and stomach flat as you do, otherwise this area will also expand as you inhale and you will not be doing Abdominal Breathing.

91

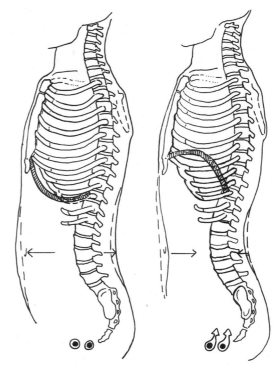

4. Fill your lungs with air. Breathe down to the diaphragm and feel it push downward.

5. The abdomen expands on all sides (not just in front) like a beach ball as you inhale. There is minimal or no expansion of the chest or stomach region above the navel.

6. When you've reached full capacity without straining yourself, pause for a second or two before exhaling.

7. Exhale slowly, contracting the abdomen with slight muscular force and simultaneously pulling up on the perineum and anus (not the sexual organs) without using too much force, as you relax the diaphragm.

8. Pause for a second or two and relax the perineum and anus before you begin the next inhalation.

9. Inhalation and exhalation should be slow and of equal length, and as silent as you can do them.

Practice for at least 5 minutes every day this week.

The Fourth Healing Sound: The Heart Sound

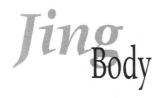

THE HEART IS ARGUABLY THE most important organ in our body, working ceaselessly to pump our blood. It is basically a large muscle in the upper left side of our chest.

Just like any other muscle, the heart is subject to the stress and tensions of everyday life. The Taoists believed that consciousness resided in the heart. The Chinese word for heart, *Hsin*, also means mind. Hsin refers to the emotional mind rather than the logical or wisdom mind which is called the Yi mind. It is easy to observe that when you are frightened the heart throbs, when you are excited it beats rapidly, when you are terrified it seems to stop, when you are hungry it feels uncomfortable, when you are facing destruction it is sad, when you are happy it is full of joy. The association of the heart with the emotional mind is not difficult to understand.

In Taoist theory, there are two hearts, the Heavenly Heart which resides in our head, between and behind the two eyes, and the heart in our chest which we are all familiar with. The Heavenly Heart is a product of our Original Essence (Yuan Jing) and our Original Energy (Yuan Chi). Our Original or Primal Spirit (Yuan Shen) resides in our Heavenly Heart which is also known as the Crystal Palace. We have already begun working in this area in the Regulating the Mind exercises.

When we are born, it is the Heavenly Heart, the Yi Mind, that rules our development. But it is our lower fleshly heart that soon usurps control, and allows us to develop, controlled by the Hsin emotional mind. This condition lasts for the rest of our lives, unless we learn to fortify and defend the Heavenly Heart—the Yi Mind—the Wisdom Mind and restore it to its rightful place as a ruler sitting on its throne, between and behind our eyes in the Square Inch Palace.

Taoist Yoga thus portrays the human heart as a rebellious organ in our body that has taken control of our nervous system and rules in place of the brain. "Ruled by your heart" is a common expression, and is a true view of the general condition of humankind. We are ruled by our emotions rather than by our intellect.

The Healing Sounds help to cool off our organs and thus restore the natural positive energy of the organ. It should be obvious that the Heart Healing Sound is the most important of all the Healing Sounds. We can build up so much heat in our hearts that it grows hard and rigid from persistent overheating.

The Heart Sound provides us with a way to gently "blow off steam," to rid our hearts of destructive heat. The Heart Sound is a precious gift preserved by Taoist sages to regulate our heart. There is no price that can be put on this piece of information. That is one reason that I'm so happy to be writing this book. These practices have been secret or unavailable for so long and they are beneficial even if you're only doing some of the exercises regularly. I intend these 100 Days of Practice to be a three-pronged approach consisting of regulating what we call the Three Treasures: the breath, the body, and the mind. I also realize that many readers will not complete, or even attempt to start, the training. That's all right. The point is you might pick out certain exercises or groups of exercises that you would like to practice. The Healing Sounds have a magical therapeutic quality of their own.

The heart is the seat of the Fire Element. The negative emotions associated with the heart are impatience, hatred, cruelty, arrogance, hastiness, violence and bigotry. How's that for a grab bag of goodies? Practically all the world's ills are somewhere on this list. All these negative, destructive emotions take root in and fester in our heart. The heat builds up. Our hearts harden. Our minds harden.

The Heart Healing Sound provides us with the means to release this heat through the fascia known as the pericardium, surrounding and regulating the temperature of the heart. The positive emotions of the heart are joy, love, learning, respect, honesty, sincerity, enthusiasm, radiance and light. Some of these reflect traditional Chinese values, especially respect. The Taoists say when you have respect the heart is open. Taoists also say that the heart provides the spirit for learning. This spirit delights in joyfulness and fun, which help provide the eagerness necessary for true learning, the kind of learning that comes from the heart.

The external organ associated with the heart is the tongue, which can move both inside and outside our mouth. The connection between the tongue and the heart may not appear obvious. But when the connection is established you will find your powers of speech improve and your ability to clear out the negative thoughts and emotions and reprogram your mind with positive energy (like this book) greatly enhanced.

The Heart Healing Sound Chi Kung is performed virtually identically to the form for the Liver Healing Sound. The only difference is you lean to the right side as you push up your interlocked fingers and the Healing Sound itself, which is H-A-W-W-W-W-W.

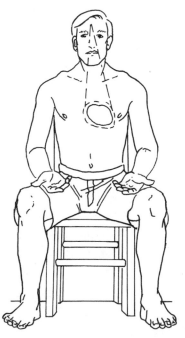

1. From a seated position, put your concentration on your heart.

2. Feel your tongue as if it were connected to your heart. Put your mind on your heart and your tongue and you will feel the connection.

3. Let your arms hang at your sides and turn your hands so that your palms face outward, away from your body.

4. Take a long deep breath as you slowly raise your arms out to your sides, palm upward. Continue raising your arms until they are overhead.

5. Look up and follow the activity above your head with your eyes.

6. Interlock the fingers of both hands overhead. Your palms now face down toward the top of your head.

7. Rotate your palms so they face upward, toward the ceiling.

8. Push up on the heel of both palms and bend from the waist a little bit to the right so that there is more of a stretch on the left side, which is the heart side.

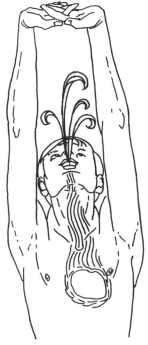

9. Open your mouth and round the lips as you exhale and silently do the Heart Sound H-A-W-W-W-W-W-W.

10. Visualize heat passing out of your heart through the surrounding fascia, the pericardium.

11. Use your imagination and bathe your heart in brilliant red light. As you exhale, the negative emotions like hatred, arrogance, cruelty and impatience exit along with the heat.

12. When you finish exhaling, disengage your fingers and slowly lower your hands and arms out to your sides.

13. Sit quietly and breathe normally for a few moments as you picture your heart surrounded by brilliant red light and filling with the positive emotions such as love, joy, respect and enthusiasm.

14. Do it at least 3 times.

The Heart Sound is also recommended for sore throats, swollen gums or tongue, any heart problems, and moodiness.

Taoist Self-Massage Rejuvenation: The Tongue

The tongue is the bridge between the body's two main Energy Channels, the Governor Channel which runs from the perineum, up the back and over the head, ending in the upper palate of the mouth and the Functional Channel which begins at the tip of the tongue and runs down the front of the body to the perineum. Raising the tip of the tongue to the roof of the mouth connects these two channels and allows the Chi to circulate continuously in the Microcosmic Orbit. However, there are many locations where the energy becomes blocked or doesn't flow freely. The tongue is one area that is highly susceptible to blockage.

There are some excellent Taoist techniques to keep the tongue strong and flexible. I'll discuss some here and some in this week's Sexual Kung Fu section.

Swallowing Saliva

This is one of the most important exercises you will learn in this book. It is used throughout the practice, from the highest to the lowest levels. The main reason is in the saliva, which has the power to lubricate the digestive glands and organs when swallowed correctly. We will be coming back to this exercise many times during the 100 Days of Practice. So let's learn it properly.

1. Place your tongue between the back of your lips and the front of your teeth, touching the upper front part of your gums.

2. Circle your tongue 9 times between the back of the lips and the front of the teeth, massaging the front upper and lower gums as you do.

3. Place the tip of your tongue behind the teeth touching the upper gums and circle the tongue 6 times in the opposite direction, massaging the upper and lower gums as you do. (It really isn't important which direction you start with, just be sure that you reverse direction when you move the tongue behind the teeth.)

4. As you circle the tongue you should find that saliva begins to flow into the mouth. This is a desired result. Move your lower jaw back and forth as if you are "chewing the saliva" for 10 to 15 seconds.

5. Raise the tip of your tongue to the upper palate just behind the teeth, and press upward with the tongue.

6. Simultaneously, pull in your chin and straighten the back of your neck which causes it to elongate as if your head were being pulled up.

7. Tighten your throat and with a gulping sound swallow the saliva, and feel it go down your throat and into the digestive organs below.

This is a hard swallow. You are forcing the saliva down your constricted throat. You will often experience all sorts of pulling and release in the throat muscles as you swallow. This is another area where we build up incredible stress and strain without usually being aware of it.

Pressing and Curling the Tongue

This is a simple exercise to strengthen the tongue and keep it flexible. The Taoists believe that strengthening the tongue also strengthens the heart.

1. Inhale, then as you exhale, stick your tongue out of your mouth and press it downward toward the ground as far as it will go.

2. Pull the tongue back into your mouth and curl it backwards, so that the tip of your tongue is facing back toward the throat.

3. Press the bottom of your tongue to the roof of your mouth as hard as you can while you simultaneously contract and pull up on the anus and tighten your throat.

4. Relax. Do exercise once or twice.

Sexual Kung Fu: Tongue Kung Fu

While we are on the subject of tongues, I decided to enlighten you with the long-time secret Taoist techniques of Tongue Kung Fu.

I first learned them in 1982 but I had suspected their existence long before that time. I know of no place else in sexual lore where these secrets have been revealed.

The Taoists often approached sex as one would approach a playing field. They would have a strategy of how best to prolong pleasure and increase the flow of Chi between the partners. The tongue played a major strategic role as one of the primary tools available to the Taoists in their quest for success on the playing field. I am not talking about seduction here. Between consenting adults, sex is seen as a playing field. As a matter of fact, many ancient Taoist sexual manuals see sex in terms of a battlefield, with its own rules of engagement and tactics to assure a satisfying outcome.

One of the most basic rules is that the woman must always climax first. I'm sure that a lot of you think this is a very good rule. There are various reasons for this rule. For one, if the man has the first orgasm, that might be the end of the battle, with the woman left not satisfied and the man falling asleep. This is not a good strategy for prolonged sex. A woman is capable of more orgasms than a man and unlike a man, won't lose Jing when she has them.

The tongue is the organ par excellence for prolonging sexual pleasure and arousal. It can change shape and size and assume an infinite variety of movements. Its surface is moist and warm with a file-like roughness. It is extremely sensitive and responsive. The tongue is also the main switch in the Microcosmic Orbit and is a powerful vehicle for passing and receiving Chi to and from your lover. It can be used by either the man or the woman in a multitude of ways, although I have to admit that it was originally conceived to be practiced by the male upon the female. But of course that was in a much less enlightened age than now.

So without any further adieu, I present the essential Tongue Kung Fu.

Note: All of the following exercises were designed to be practiced with a partner. If you have no partner available, it is suggested that you hang a piece of fruit, such as an orange, from a string by tying a toothpick to the string and embedding one end of the toothpick one inch into the orange. Hang the fruit at mouth level and practice as below. When you have mastered the orange, you can proceed to the grapefruit.

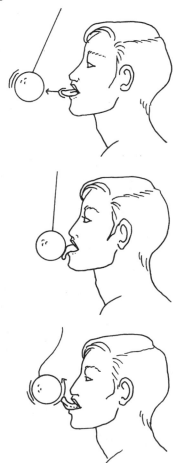

1. *The Serpent Tongue:* Lash out with your tongue like a snake. Project it quickly out of the mouth, making it firm and sharp-pointed. Shoot it straight forward and practice increasing speed. The Serpent Tongue is recommended for stimulating your partner's ears, breasts (nipples) and genitals.

2. *The Hook Tongue:* In this esoteric practice, you stick your tongue out and down toward your chin, then hook it upward and lick upward with the tip of the tongue. Repeated experiments by dedicated Taoists over thousands of years have clearly shown that this form of Tongue Kung Fu is especially stimulating to the genitals of both sexes.

3. *The Slap Tongue:* Stick the tongue out and bring it to the left side of the mouth. Quickly swing the outstretched tongue to the right side of the mouth, slapping anything that might be in its way. Repeat from right to left, etc. As you practice you will find your slap increasing in speed and power. This

form of Tongue Kung Fu has also been shown to be an effective means of genital arousal for members of both sexes. Use this one to increase your tongue's agility and nimbleness.

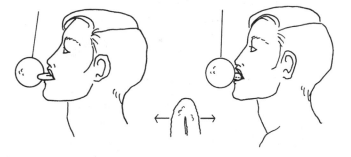

4. *The Drill Tongue:* This secret practice was developed to deal with the problem of tumescent (erect) nipples. The tip of the tongue is used to push the protruding nipple back into the breast. Once it is pushed back, the tip of the tongue is used to whirl the nipple around in little circles. Taoist sages found this created a thrilling spiral of energy for their partners.

There is no substitute for practice here. Experiment and find new and exciting uses for Tongue Kung Fu. A little practice goes a long way. There are a couple of additional rules:

    a. Observe reasonable standards of hygiene, i.e., wash.

    b. When performing Tongue Kung Fu on the genitals, use the tip of one finger to seal the opening of your partner's anus. This prevents the loss of Chi which is easily leaked out during arousal.

These are authentic Taoist practices. As you can see, the Taoists thought of everything.

Baduanjin: The Seventh and Eighth Pieces

This week we learn the final two Pieces of the Brocade. These last two are probably the easiest to learn of all the Pieces.

These eight exercises are an excellent way to get started in the morning. You can probably do all eight of them the recommended eight times within five minutes. They are also good any other time you need to loosen up. They are among the most well known of all the forms of Chi Kung. Do them all this week. After this week I will continue teaching you new exercises, but you should not forget the Eight Pieces of Brocade. Try to do them every day.

The Seventh Piece:
Clenching the Fists and Glaring to Increase Strength

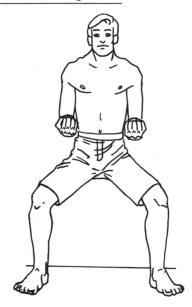

1. Stand with feet wide apart as in Second Piece: Drawing the Bow on Both Sides. Bend the knees as if riding a horse while keeping the back straight.

2. Form each hand into a fist and bring each fist to the side of the body next to the waist. Palm side of fist faces upward and knuckle side of fist faces downward.

3. Slowly thrust the right fist out to the right side. As you do this, turn the fist over so that when the right arm is fully extended, the palm side of the fist faces downward.

4. Open both eyes wide, glaring toward the moving fist.

5. Return the right fist to starting position.

6. Slowly thrust the left fist out to the left side. As you do this, turn the fist over so that when the left arm is fully extended, the palm side of the fist faces downward and knuckles face upward.

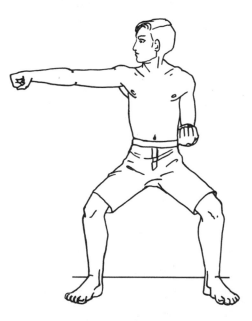

7. Return the left fist to starting position at the waist.

8. Exhale when thrusting out with fist and inhale when returning fist to side.

9. Do 8 times on each side.

In this Piece, it is necessary that the fists be firmly clenched. Grip the ground with your toes. Thrust out the arms slowly using the strength of the whole body; this is not the same as throwing a quick punch. Your mind must be concentrated on the exercise and the eyes must glare as if angry to enhance blood circulation, stimulate the iris, cerebral cortex and autonomic nervous system. Glaring is an important part of the exercise. It helps to reinforce the strength of the clenched fist. Continued practice with this exercise will promote muscular development and increase body strength and endurance.

The Eighth Piece: Raising and Lowering the Heels to Jolt the Body and Cure All Illnesses

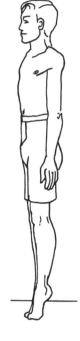

1. Stand at attention with feet together or no more than a few inches apart. Keep the open palms hanging loosely by the sides and keep the legs straight.

2. Raise both heels off the ground simultaneously, so that you are balanced on the toes. Your eyes look straight ahead or slightly upward.

3. Quickly drop both heels to the ground, jolting the entire body.

4. Inhale as you raise the heels and exhale as you lower them.

5. Repeat 8 times.

This final Piece sets off a light vibration in the entire body, which serves as a perfect final touch for the entire set of Baduanjin.

Warming the Stove

YOU ARE NOW FOUR WEEKS into the practice. If you have been practicing these Regulating the Mind exercises regularly, you should be getting some interesting results. You might have realized, by what I've written earlier in this chapter about the Hsin-Emotional and Yi-Wisdom Mind, that the Third Treasure practices are designed to stimulate the Yi Mind, the Higher Mind.

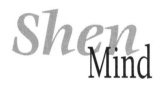

Last week we ended the session by directing our consciousness three inches behind the Third Eye Point, which lies between and just slightly above the two eyes. This area is the location of the Heavenly Heart, also called the Crystal Palace, Upper Tan Tien or Cavity of Original Spirit.

As you've seen through the various Three Treasure exercises in this book, connecting or feeling, sensing, imagining or visualizing a connection between different parts of the body is a crucial part of Taoist Yoga and Chi Kung.

It's time now to learn a connection that is basically unknown in the West, but is a key to the true practice. To do this I will again have to provide more theory so that the meditation makes sense.

While we were floating in our mother's womb, we were attached to her by the umbilical cord. Jing from our mother entered our body through the umbilical cord and was stored behind the umbilicus in the Ocean of Chi. A central part of this Ocean of Chi is the Tan Tien, or more correctly the Lower Tan Tien. It is this place, our Lower Tan Tien, that we want to connect to the Upper Tan Tien behind the mid-eye point.

The Lower Tan Tien's exact location is different in each person, but it is generally located two finger widths or 1.3 inches below your navel and between halfway to two-thirds of the way inside, between your navel and your back, i.e., closer to your spine than your navel. To the fledgling Taoist, this is the most important place in the body. Be aware, though, that many Chinese texts give different locations for the Tan Tien, some three inches below the navel and some closer to the front of the body. For the exercises in this book, use the position I give. Later on, when you learn the Microcosmic Orbit, we will also use the navel point as the Tan Tien.

Tan Tien translates as "Elixir Field." An elixir is a healing medicine or potion, so we can also translate Tan Tien as "Medicine Field." This gives us a hint of the practice and part of the secret of the Golden Flower.

The Lower Tan Tien is where Jing-Essence is converted into Chi. This restores our Original Chi-Yuan Chi. This Original Chi is the Elixir or Medicine.

In theory it's all very simple. The Taoists sought to restore the Original Energy that existed in us when we were first born. This Original Energy kept us healthy and ensured the free flow of Vital Life Force Energy, another name for Original Chi, throughout our entire body. The Taoists believe that restoration of the Original Chi will restore perfect health to the body.

The process begins by lowering your concentration into the Lower Tan Tien, like a plumb line, from the Upper Tan Tien above at the Third Eye Point. The Elixir is prepared by warming up the Lower Tan Tien using rapid Abdominal Breathing. We call this breathing Bellows Breathing.

In Bellows Breathing you inhale and expand the abdomen rapidly and forcefully. You exhale rapidly and forcefully. An inhalation and exhalation should take no more than a second. The Breath is seen as the old blacksmith tool the bellows, which is used to raise the heat of the blacksmith's fire. This accounts for its other name, Quick Fire. We can also now see why the Lower Tan Tien was also referred to as the Stove. The Bellows Breathing raises the temperature of the Stove and hence the name of this week's practice, "Warming the Stove."

These Regulation of the Mind – Third Treasure exercises build upon each other week by week. I won't repeat the details from the previous week's exercise, to save this book from being any more tedious and long-winded than necessary. However, I will tell you what part of the previous week's exercise should be done first before doing the new material. It is most important to continue practicing the basic exercises. We are building a firm foundation here. I commend you if you have read this far and kept up with the practice. Your persistence will be rewarded.

1. Repeat last week's Regulating the Mind exercise up to the point where you have smiled into the various parts of your eyes and connected the smile to a smile on the raised corner of your lips. Once you have connected the left and right outer and inner corners of the eyes, the pupils, the irises, the whites and the upper and lower eyelids, we are ready to pick up this week's exercise.

2. Feel your whole left eye smiling and feel the connection with the raised left corner of your lips. Feel the outer corner of your left eye crinkle up as you smile.

3. Feel your whole right eye smiling and feel the connection with the raised right corner of your lips. Feel the outer corner of your right eye crinkle up as you smile.

4. Quickly transfer your concentration to the tip of your nose and raise it fairly rapidly to the "bump" and then the Third Eye Point, between and slightly above the two eyes.

5. Smile into the Third Eye point. Sense this smile move into the space behind the Third Eye, as if you could turn your eyesight around and look into your head. Remain here for 2 minutes or more.

6. Place your tongue between the front of your teeth and the back of your lips and circle 9 times in either direction, then place tongue behind the teeth and circle 6 times in the opposite direction. Your mouth should fill with saliva. Move your lower jaw forward and back as if you were "chewing the saliva" as you smile into the saliva.

7. Place the tip of your tongue to the roof of your mouth behind the teeth. Pull in your chin, straighten the back of the neck and tighten your throat and swallow the saliva with a gulping sound.

8. Follow the path of the saliva and lower your concentration, and the smiling energy, to the spot approximately two-thirds of the way inside your body and a little more than an inch below your navel, to the Lower Tan Tien. If you can sense or feel nothing, just use your imagination and estimate where it should be.

9. Do 18 or more Bellow Breaths, which are short, rapid Abdominal Breaths of no more than one second duration for each inhalation and exhalation. Use the abdominal muscles to forcefully contract the abdomen on exhalation. Inhale and exhale through the nose.

10. The Lower Tan Tien should start to feel warm. It may take a few days or even a few weeks to experience this, but if you practice it will warm up. Keep your concentration on the Lower Tan Tien for a few minutes as we now switch to slow Abdominal Breathing (this is called Slow Fire).

11. To finish the exercise:

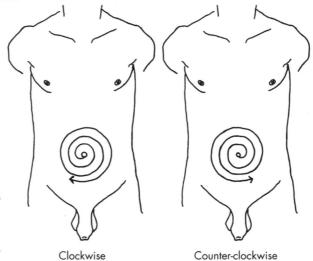

Clockwise   Counter-clockwise

Men: Put your left hand over your navel, cover it with your right hand. Circle the navel, in 3-inch circles, with the two palms over each other, 36 times clockwise (from above down on the left side and come up on the right side) and then reverse 24 times counterclockwise. Use your mind as well to guide the Chi around the navel. On the final circulation draw the Chi into the Lower Tan Tien.

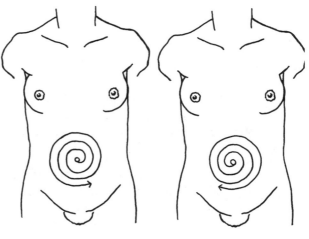

Counter-clockwise   Clockwise

Women: Put your right hand over your navel and cover it with your left hand. Circle the navel, in 3-inch circles, with the two palms over each other, 36 times counter-clockwise (from above down on the right side and come up on the left side) and then reverse 24 times clockwise. Use your mind as well to guide the Chi around the navel. On the final circulation draw the Chi into the Lower Tan Tien.

12. Rub your palms together until hot and Massage the Face. Rub them again and cover the eyes and absorb the Chi into your eyes.

You learn some new and important techniques here. In step 11 we learn to collect Energy into the Lower Tan Tien. This will become the standard way to close the Regulating the Mind exercises for the rest of the 100 Days of Practice.

Some people will feel heat in the Lower Tan Tien almost immediately. For others it will take some time. That is part of the difficulty in putting a book like this together. Some of you will excel in certain areas and some in others. I wish I could be there with each one of you to offer personal guidance. If you feel nothing, just do the exercises daily then move on to Week Five. We will continue Warming the Stove as we learn the Inner Smile over the next three weeks. By the end of four weeks of practice you should be experiencing warmth in and around or behind the navel area. Don't get anxious or press for results. They will come in time. Anxiety about your progress will hamper your progress. All you have to feel is some warmth in the lower abdomen. Feel secure in the fact that sooner or later you will.

week five

THIS WEEK WE FINISH THE first and begin the second month of the 100 Days of Practice. I hope you have enjoyed the material up to now. I have tried my best to keep my lessons as simple and coherent as possible. I certainly encourage you to go back and review what you've already learned. It's all necessary to build the firm foundation required for success with the 100 Days of Practice.

As you can see, the Taoist approach to health, rejuvenation, longevity and sex is logical, novel and creative. There is a refreshing blend of a highly serious discipline with a somewhat irreverent point of view.

You now know a lot of exercises, and the Healing Sounds, Taoist Self-Massage Rejuvenation, the Eight Pieces of Brocade and the Sexual Kung Fu can be practiced every day. You don't have to do all of the old material and all the new material every day. I've given you enough so you can pick and choose. One word of advice: if there is any type or group of exercises that you have been ignoring, chances are these are the ones you need to do most.

Abdominal Breathing and Perineum Power: Part Two

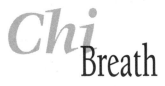

THIS WEEK'S REGULATING THE BREATH exercise will be a variation of last week's exercise. Last week we learned Abdominal Breathing combining pulling up on the perineum and anus when we exhaled.

This week we will continue to strengthen and increase our awareness of the perineum area. We will continue to do the inhalation as before. On the exhalation we will alternate between pulling up only the perineum muscle and not the anus on one exhalation and pulling up only on the anus and not on the perineum on the next exhalation.

I can't emphasize enough the importance of strengthening the perineum area. Our entire body rests on top of the perineum every time we are upright. If this area is weak, it has a profound effect on the rest of our body; we will constantly be leaking energy. When the area is strengthened, we build up Perineum Power, which not only strengthens the perineum but becomes increasingly important in terms of our ability to direct Chi up and down the Governor and Functional Channels.

1. Do an Abdominal Breath inhalation expanding the lower abdomen.

2. Exhale and contract the abdominal muscles as you simultaneously pull up only on the perineum (Hui Yin), located between the back of the sexual organs and the front of the anus. Do not pull up on the anus itself or the sexual organs.

3. Relax the perineum and do another Abdominal Breath inhalation, expanding the lower abdomen on all sides.

4. Exhale and contract the abdominal muscles as you simultaneously pull up only on the anus. Do not pull up the perineum itself or the sexual organs.

5. Relax the anus as you do the next inhalation.

6. Practice at least 5 minutes every day, alternating between pulling up on the perineum on one exhalation and the anus on the next.

The Fifth Healing Sound: The Spleen Sound

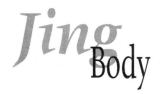

THE SPLEEN IS PROBABLY THE least well known of the five Taoist major internal organs. The Taoists believe the spleen produces antibodies to protect us against certain diseases. This function is not fully recognized in the West, where the full function of the spleen is still somewhat of a mystery. As opposed to the other four major organs, loss of the spleen will not necessarily do any serious damage to the body. The spleen does function to remove worn-out red and white blood cells and break down hemoglobin and acts as a reservoir for iron in our body. In the fetal stage and shortly after birth, the spleen produces all sorts of blood cells, but by our ninth month most of this function is taken over by the bone marrow, with the spleen producing white blood cells known as lymphocytes.

The spleen is located on the left side of the body at the top of the abdominal cavity. It is a soft oval-shaped organ. The spleen lies in direct contact with the pancreas which runs across the middle of the body, on a line from the liver to the spleen. The pancreas is vital to our body's existence. It produces the insulin that regulates our blood sugar level. In the absence of sufficient insulin, our blood sugar level rises to toxic levels, which is basically what happens if you have diabetes mellitus. Excess insulin leads to the condition known as hypoglycemia, which can also be fatal unless controlled.

The Taoists perceived an intimate relationship between the spleen and the pancreas. Very often the organ is referred to as the spleen/pancreas. The Healing Sound works on both organs. The Sound is W-H-O-O-O-O-O, like an owl.

The exterior organ of the spleen is the mouth, especially the lips. Some old sources include the flesh of the entire face as the exterior organ of the spleen.

The Element of the spleen is the Earth Element. The negative emotion of the spleen is worry and self-pity. Its positive emotions or qualities are openness and fairness to yourself and others.

1. Sit up in a chair with your legs wide apart. Your hands rest on the middle of your thighs, palm side upward.

2. Become aware of your spleen on the left upper side of your abdomen at the bottom of the ribcage as well as your pancreas which runs across the center of your body at the level of your stomach.

3. Inhale a deep or Abdominal Breath and raise your hands and press the index, middle and ring fingers of both hands into the solar plexus area, about 1-1/2 to 2 inches below the sternum (breastbone).

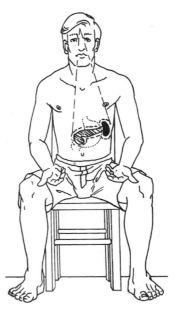

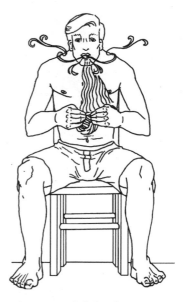

4. Exhale as you press into the solar plexus area and subvocally make the Healing Sound W-H-O-O-O-O-O-O.

5. Bend slightly forward as you finish the exhalation.

6. Use your imagination or feel excess heat escaping from the spleen and solar plexus area. Imagine that worry and self-pity are being expelled from the spleen/pancreas as you exhale and make the Healing Sound W-H-O-O-O-O-O-O.

7. Sit up straight and lower your palms into your lap as you return to the starting position.

8. Sit quietly and breathe normally and imagine the area of the spleen, stomach, solar plexus and pancreas bathed in a bright yellow or golden yellow light. Feel or imagine the qualities of openness and fairness filling this entire area. (Openness is the ability to be open to new ideas, people or experiences.)

9. Repeat at least 3 times per session.

Taoist Self-Massage Rejuvenation

The mouth is the external organ of the spleen. In this week's Taoist Self-Massage Rejuvenation exercises, we will concentrate on exercises for the mouth and teeth.

Clicking the Teeth Together

This is one of the best known of the self-massage techniques and is often taught as part of Sitting Baduanjin. The exercise couldn't be simpler. You just click your teeth together. Often the clicking was followed by Swallowing Saliva in the Taoist fashion as taught last week. The clicking helps to keep the teeth strong and prevents gum disease. Also it sets up a light vibration that reverberates through the bones of the jaw and skull and helps to relieve tension in these areas. Clicking the Teeth Together should be done every day.

1. Click the back teeth together approximately 18 times.

2. Click the front teeth together approximately 18 times.

3. If you have the time, or the inclination, Swallow Saliva.

Tapping the Gums

This is another simple exercise to keep the gums healthy.

1. Rub your hands together until hot.

2. Using the index, middle and ring fingers of either hand, tap the gums around the upper and lower teeth, moving in an oval-shaped pattern. Tap on the outside of the mouth around the lips, not inside the mouth.

Beautify the Mouth Massage

This exercise will help you when practicing the Smiling exercises you learned in Week Three. The exercise also stands on its own as a means to beautify the mouth.

Appearance often tells us a lot about a person. The expression on someone's face can help to inform us whether that person is happy or sad. Sadness, stress, and depression cause the muscles of the mouth to loosen and lose their natural tone. This leads to a slackness at the corners of the mouth which sag and drop and gives the face a sad or depressed appearance.

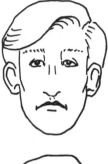

Looking cheerful and happy is much more attractive and depends to quite an extent on the corners of the lips and the eyes. Massaging the mouth muscles will help to lift up the corners of your mouth. When the corners are lifted, your cheeks also rise up and your whole face seems to be filled with more positive energy. Connecting this energy with smiling eyes has a radiant effect on your face and makes you feel much happier. Try it. With a little practice, people will quickly take notice.

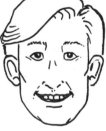

1. Rub your hands together until hot.

2. Raise the thumb and index finger of your right hand to both corners of the lips.

3. Feel the Chi pass from the thumb and index fingers into the corners of the mouth.

4. Press in a little and raise up the corners of the lips, toward the eyes, about 1 inch.

5. Release.

6. Do 10 to 20 times every day.

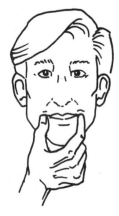

Chi Kung

Over the years, I've had the opportunity to learn from and observe many teachers and practitioners of Chi Kung. There are many different forms and styles. One teacher from mainland China tells me that he knows over two hundred different forms. Mantak Chia told me that what's really important is to master some basic forms and learn to build a firm foundation in controlling the Chi. He said those who never build a firm foundation just keep learning more and more forms of Chi Kung and Tai Chi and actually move further away from following the Way as they delude themselves into thinking they are making progress with the Tao.

Personally I enjoy learning new forms every once in a while. However, I try not to learn too many different forms within a short timeframe because there is just too much to practice. If I practiced everything I know, I'd be at it twenty-four hours a day. There is absolutely no need for this. I said when we started the practice that only fifteen minutes of your time was necessary every day. By this week, you may be finding yourself devoting a half hour or more a day. Still, this is not a lot of time. Although I've given you many things to do, after you've gotten past learning each week's exercises, they really don't take very long to perform. What is important is to practice every day.

There are hard forms of Chi Kung performed by seasoned martial artists, such as the ability to absorb what would otherwise be a deadly blow to the body, which are beyond the scope of this book. There are the moderate forms like the Eight Pieces of Brocade that seek to move your Energy by combining breathing with movement. There are also soft forms which are concerned with sensing and controlling the flow of Chi. These forms require little or no movement and often involve the ability to absorb and transmit Chi into and out of the fingers and palms of the hands. This branch of Chi Kung is often associated with healing. We will learn some basics this week.

Activating the Palms and Fingertips – Holding the Chi Ball

1. Rub your hands together until hot.

2. Keeping the palms in contact, bring the two hands in front of you at the level of your heart.

3. Slowly separate your hands until your palms are about an inch apart. Your fingers should be slightly curved toward each other with the fingertips almost touching.

4. Concentrate on a point in between the two palms with both your eyes and your mind. This will cause Chi to flow into the palms and fingertips.

5. Feel a ball of Energy develop between your
   hands. You might sense a tingling sensation, or a
   sense of heat expanding or an Energy web that is
   difficult to describe with words. You should feel
   something in the "empty" space between your
   two hands.

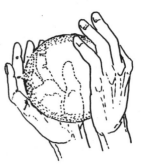

6. Slowly move the hands farther apart until the
   space between the palms is about four to five
   inches, with the fingers still curved toward each
   other. Use your mind to feel or sense the Chi
   Ball grow bigger.

7. Move the hands in and out a few times. If you continue to pull the
   palms farther apart, you will reach a point where you will lose the
   energetic connection between the palms. This point is different for
   everybody and depends on a number of variables each day. So experiment and find out how far you can move the palms and fingertips
   apart before you lose the Chi Ball.

8. Move your hands closer together and sense or feel the Chi Ball
   condense.

9. Play with the Chi Ball. Circle the fingertips around each other and feel
   the ball of radiating Chi seem to push your two hands apart.

10. Maintaining the Chi Ball between the palms, move the palms in uni-
    son upward, then downward, to the left and finally to the right.

11. Return to the original position and pull the palms apart and then
    move them closer together a few times.

12. To close: from a sitting position, rest your hands in your lap, palms
    facing upward, and feel or imagine that as you inhale you are drawing
    Chi into the center of your palms and as you exhale you expel Chi
    from this same spot, as if your palms were breathing. Do this for at
    least 30 seconds.

    From a standing position, move the palms apart and turn them so
    they are facing upward and imagine or feel that as you inhale you are
    drawing Chi into the center of your palm and as you exhale you are
    expelling Chi from this same spot. Do this for 30 seconds or more.

One of the maxims of Taoist belief is that blood follows Chi. This means
that when you direct and gather Chi in a certain place in your body, you also
increase the flow of blood to that same spot. The fingertips are connected to
many Energy Meridians in the body. Gathering Chi into the fingers and palms
activates Chi in our organs and glands and improves blood circulation to these

same organs and glands. This is one reason that so many of these exercises begin by rubbing the two hands together. You've probably heard that cold hands are a sign of poor circulation. The Taoists believed this. If you suffer from cold hands, now you have the means to overcome this condition. By the way, if you have normally warm hands, it might initially reduce your ability to sense or feel the Chi Ball. Practice makes perfect.

Yin-Yang Palm

This exercise extends the concept of "breathing" in and out of our palms as taught in the last exercise. The Taoists believed that the palms could be trained to absorb Chi from the universe (Heavenly Chi) and transmit it to the world around us.

In the Taoist scheme of things, the entire manifest universe is ruled by three original forces, the Three Pure Ones. These Three Pure Ones were brought into existence through the interaction of Yin and Yang. The Taoist classic, *Tao Te Ching* of Lao Tzu, tells us that:

> *The Tao produced the One (Tai Chi);*
> *The One produced the Two (Yin and Yang);*
> *The Two produced the Three (The Three Pure Ones);*
> *The Three produced all the myriad beings (all of existence).*

The Three Pure Ones are one, *Universal* or *Heavenly Chi*; two, *Human Plane Chi*; and three, *Earth Chi*. Heavenly Chi includes the Chi or Energy of all the planets, stars and constellations as well as the Energy of God (the force of creation and universal love). Human Plane Chi is the Energy that exists on the surface of our planet and sustains human life and the Earth force includes all of the forces inside the planet as well as the Five Elemental Forces.

In this exercise we connect ourselves, the Human Plane, with the Heavenly Force from above and the Earth Force below. To accomplish this we absorb Heavenly Chi into our left palm, the Yin Palm, and transmit it into the Earth with our right palm, the Yang Palm. Earlier when I described Yin and Yang, I said we would be most concerned with their aspects of being receptive (Yin) and active (Yang). Our left palm receives Heavenly Chi and is thus Yin, while our right palm is active and transmits Chi into the Earth and is therefore Yang.

Yin-Yang Palm is a simple, peaceful practice that is always enhanced by smiling energy.

1. Sit up straight in a chair and close your eyes and establish smiling energy in your eyes and feel the connection with the corners of your mouth.

2. Your left hand rests on your left thigh, fingers open and palm facing upward toward the sky.

3. Your right hand is held next to your right thigh, with fingers open and your palm facing down toward the ground.

4. Imagine that as you inhale Chi is spiraling clockwise down from above and entering the center of your left palm.

5. The Chi moves up your left arm to your shoulder and across your chest to your right shoulder.

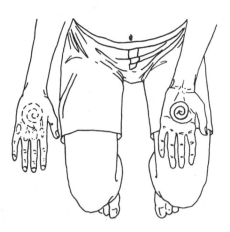

6. When you exhale, Chi is emitted from the center of your right palm and spirals counterclockwise down into the Earth.

7. Continue for a few minutes.

8. To complete, rub your hands together and massage your face.

This exercise forms the basis of many Taoist healing techniques, where the right palm is used to transmit healing Chi into yourself or others. This is a highly developed art form in China. The transmission of Chi is accepted as scientifically correct and is practiced by Chinese medical doctors. Please note that the Chi that is transmitted is first absorbed from outside the practitioner, so that he or she acts as a conduit for the energy, rather than transmitting one's own energy, which is considered to be highly dangerous and potentially debilitating.

Sexual Kung Fu

In Week Three we learned how to increase our production of Jing Chi—Sexual Energy. Last Week we learned Tongue Kung Fu which is a part of the vast treasury of Taoist lovemaking techniques designed to ultimately balance male and female Sexual Energy. This week we turn our attention to the conservation of Sexual Energy.

I have mentioned numerous times that men lose Jing Chi through ejaculation and women lose Jing Chi during menstruation. These are the main ways that Sexual Energy is lost by either sex. We also lose Jing Chi if our sexual organs are weak.

Both men and women have two "gates" in their sexual organs that allow Jing Chi to leak out if they are not properly toned. This week's exercise, Closing the Two Front Gates, will teach you where these gates are located and how to strengthen them. Because of the difference in anatomy between men and women, the description of the exercise is somewhat different for each although the practice is basically the same.

Closing the Two Front Gates

Men: The first gate is located in the opening at the tip of the penis. If you put your concentration here, you can close off the opening. The second gate is located at the base of the penis, where it is attached to the body. Just behind this point is the urogenital diaphragm. If you put your concentration here, you can close this gate as well by contracting the urogenital diaphragm.

1. Lightly contract the gate at the tip of the penis.

2. Contract the gate at the base of the penis (urogenital diaphragm).

3. Simultaneously pull in on the eye muscles. If you can, pay special attention to the circular muscles of the iris and pull in on these as well as the muscles surrounding the eye.

4. Do this 3 to 9 times.

5. You do not have to coordinate this exercise with breathing, but you can if you want to. Experiment with pulling up on the inhalation and then with pulling up on the exhalation. Which way feels stronger to you?

Urogenital diaphragm
(Second Gate)

Tip of Penis
(First Gate)

Women: The first gate is the opening of the vagina. Concentrate on the opening of the lips of the vagina and contract them. The second gate lies inside the vagina at the urogenital diaphragm in front of the opening to the cervix. If you concentrate here, you can contract this point.

1. Lightly contract the gate at the lips of the vagina.

2. Contract the gate inside the vagina at the urogenital diaphragm.

3. Simultaneously pull in on the eye muscles. If you can, pay special attention to the circular muscles of the iris and pull in on these as well as the muscles surrounding the eye.

4. Do this 3 to 9 times.

5. You do not have to coordinate this exercise with breathing, but you can if you want to. Experiment with pulling up on the inhalation and then with pulling up on the exhalation. Which way feels stronger to you?

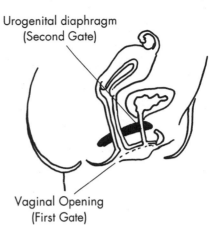

Urogenital diaphragm
(Second Gate)

Vaginal Opening
(First Gate)

Men and Women: If you have any difficulty locating the second gate here is another exercise that also works well to strengthen this gate.

When you urinate, try to stop the flow of urine by squeezing deep inside your penis or vagina. The place you have to squeeze to stop the flow is the location of the second gate. Squeezing the first gate at the tip of the penis or lips of the vagina is unlikely to stop the flow by itself.

The Inner Smile: The Front Line

WE HAVE ALREADY LEARNED how to smile into our eyes. We also learned how to smile into the Third Eye and smile into the saliva in our mouth before swallowing it and following the smile as it descended down into the Tan Tien.

Shen **Mind**

This week we will continue the process of turning the smile around, and learn how to smile into our body's five major organs. Smiling into our organs is an excellent way to put us directly in contact with what is going on inside of us.

You should already know the locations of the five major organs.

The Inner Smile is a uniquely Taoist technique that works on a whole bunch of levels. The Inner Smile begins in the eyes. The eyes are connected to our autonomic (involuntary) nervous system which in turn is connected to all of our organs and glands. Our eyes receive visual impulses which are interpreted as emotional signals which cause our organs and glands to increase activity in times of stress or danger and slow down when things get more peaceful. Ideally, the eyes should maintain a calm and balanced level of response to stimuli.

The Inner Smile works as a powerful relaxation technique as you learn to send smiling, loving energy directly into our five major organs that the Taoists believe control our emotional states. An Inner Smile directed into our organs and glands also has the power to heal, repair and rejuvenate them and help them to function optimally.

1. Repeat step 1 of last week's Regulating the Mind exercise and visualize a smiling Sun or Moon. Smile into the various parts of your eyes and connect the smile to a smile on the raised corner of your lips. Connect the left and right outer and inner corners of the eyes, the pupils, the irises, the whites and the upper and lower eyelids.

2. Feel your whole left eye smiling and feel the connection with the raised left corner of your lips. Feel the outer corner of your left eye crinkle up as you smile.

3. Feel your whole right eye smiling and feel the connection with the raised right corner of your lips. Feel the outer corner of your right eye crinkle up as you smile.

4. Feel both eyes smiling.

5. Smile into the Third Eye point. Feel this smile radiate down your nose and from there, spread out into your face. Smile into your cheeks and your ears.

6. Raise the tip of your tongue to the roof of your mouth. Keep it there for the remainder of this exercise.

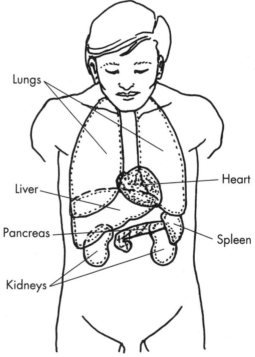

7. Re-establish the smile in your Third Eye and feel it descend to the roof of your mouth. Feel the tension in the roof of your mouth dissolve as you smile into it.

8. The smile descends down your tongue and into your throat. Feel your head sinking down into your chest, like a turtle's head.

9. Smile into your heart. Feel your heart smile. Fill your heart with smiling, loving energy. Thank your heart for beating and pumping blood to all parts of your body and keeping you alive.

10. Smile into your lungs. Say hello to your lungs and thank them for breathing and keeping you alive.

11. Smile into your liver. A real smile. Thank your liver for performing its numerous functions that help to keep you alive.

12. Smile into your two kidneys. Fill both kidneys with smiling, loving energy. Thank your kidneys for removing liquid waste and for keeping you alive.

13. Smile into your spleen and pancreas. Say hello to both and thank them for keeping you alive.

14. Reestablish the smile in your Third Eye point. Sense this smile move into the space behind the Third Eye, as if you could turn your eyesight around and look into your head. Remain here for a minute or two.

15. Place your tongue between the front of your teeth and the back of your lips and circle 9 times in either direction, then place tongue behind the teeth and circle 6 times in the opposite direction. Your mouth should fill with saliva. Move your lower jaw forward and back as if you were "chewing the saliva" as you smile into the saliva.

16. Place the tip of your tongue to the roof of your mouth behind the teeth. Pull in your chin, straighten the back of the neck and tighten your throat and swallow the saliva with a gulping sound.

17. Follow the path of the saliva and lower your concentration, and the smiling energy, to the spot two-thirds of the way inside your body and a little more than an inch below your navel, to the Lower Tan Tien. If you can sense or feel nothing, just use your imagination and estimate where it should be.

18. Do 18 or more Bellows Breaths, which are short, rapid Abdominal Breaths of no more than one second duration for each inhalation and exhalation. Use the abdominal muscles to forcefully contract the abdomen on exhalation. Inhale and exhale through the nose.

19. The Lower Tan Tien should start to feel warm. Listen to your breathing and keep your concentration on the Lower Tan Tien for a few minutes and do slow Abdominal Breathing (Slow Fire).

20. To finish the exercise:

    Men: Put your left hand over your navel, cover it with your right hand. Circle the navel, in 3-inch circles, with the two palms over each other, 36 times clockwise (from above down on the left side and come up on the right side) and then reverse 24 times counterclockwise. Use your mind as well to guide the Chi around the navel. On the final circulation draw the Chi into the Lower Tan Tien.

    Women: Put your right hand over your navel and cover it with your left hand. Circle the navel, in 3-inch circles, with the two palms over each other, 36 times counter-clockwise (from above down on the right side and come up on the left side) and then reverse 24 times clockwise. Use your mind as well to guide the Chi around the navel. On the final circulation draw the Chi into the Lower Tan Tien.

21. Rub your palms together until hot and Massage the Face. Rub them again and cover the eyes and absorb the Chi into your eyes.

Perineum Power and Sexual Kung Fu

AS WE MOVE DEEPER INTO the practice of Taoist Yoga, it becomes more difficult to teach exercises that don't combine Regulating the Breath and Regulating the Body. As I previously mentioned, there are very few "pure" breathing exercises. Breathing affects the rest of
your body. When you inhale air, the oxygen in the air is absorbed into your bloodstream in your lungs and from there is transported by your circulatory system to every living cell in your body. There is an intimate relationship within our body of our First Treasure, Chi, with our Second Treasure, Jing.

You have been practicing Abdominal Breathing since Week Two. Last week you learned to alternately pull up on the perineum on one exhalation and the anus on the next. You also learned how to Close the Two Front Gates of the sexual organs.

This week we will learn how to take an even deeper breath and really increase our intake of air. To accomplish this we will take an inhalation and expand our abdomen and lower lungs. We will then shift our attention upward as we continue to inhale and fill the middle of our lungs. When the middle of the lungs are full, we shift our attention to the top of the lungs and inhale a little more to completely fill our lungs. You should feel fully packed.

We will then exhale in the reverse order in which we inhaled. We exhale from the upper lungs first, then the middle lungs and finally the lower abdomen.

As we exhale from our upper lungs, we will pull up only on our sexual organs. As we exhale from the middle of our lungs, we also pull up on our perineum. Finally as we exhale from our lower abdomen, we pull up on our anus as well.

This exercise continues the process of learning to distinguish and differentiate between the various parts of the perineum area. As you perform it you may feel you are drawing Sexual Energy backward from the sexual organs toward the perineum and finally the anus. In future lessons we will learn to continue drawing this Jing Chi into and up the spine. This process of reversing the directional flow of Sexual Energy from outward to backward is also called the Backward Flowing Method in *The Secret of the Golden Flower*. This term is also applied to the method of turning the eyesight from outward to inward as you've been learning in the Regulating the Mind sections since Week One.

1. This exercise can be done standing, sitting or lying down.

2. Do an Abdominal Breath and fill and expand the lower abdomen.

3. Continue inhaling, shifting your attention upward, slightly expanding the lower rib cage as you completely fill the lower and middle part of the lungs.

4. Continue inhaling and raise your attention to the top of your lungs and fill the upper region of the lungs with air. Don't inhale so much that it is uncomfortable or painful, but you should feel pretty full and expanded. In all likelihood, you have rarely taken this much air into your system at one time. Initially it might feel strange or you might get lightheaded. If this happens cut back on the air intake a little until you are more comfortable with this exercise.

5. Pause for a second or two and then begin exhaling from the upper lungs only. Simultaneously pull up on your sexual organs, Closing the Two Front Gates, as you learned last week. Men should also pull up on the testicles. Hold on to the pull; do not release it until the entire exhalation is finished.

6. Pause for a second and then exhale from the middle and lower lungs as you simultaneously pull up on the perineum. Hold the pull through the next two steps so that you are now pulling up on the perineum and the sexual organs.

7. Pause for a second and exhale and contract the lower abdomen as you simultaneously pull up on the anus.

8. Hold the pull on the anus, perineum and sexual organs for a second or two and then release.

9. Do at least 3 times at first few sessions then increase to 6 or more per session.

The Sixth Healing Sound: The Triple Warmer Sound

THE TRIPLE WARMER IS NOT an organ as we understand organs in the West. Rather it refers to what the Taoists saw as three regions in the body: the upper region, the middle region and the lower region. As you descend from the head down through the body, the upper 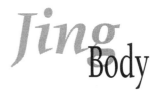 region is considered to be hot, the middle region to be warm and the lower region to be cool. The upper region consists of the brains, the heart and the lungs. The middle region comprises the kidneys, liver, spleen, pancreas and stomach. The lower region includes the entire lower abdomen, the large and small intestines, the sexual organs and the bladder.

The Triple Warmer Sound is used to regulate and balance the temperature in these three regions of the body. You imagine or feel energy rolling down your body from your head to your lower abdomen as you make the Healing Sound. Hot energy is brought down to the lower regions and cold energy rises up through the digestive system to balance out the temperature in the three regions.

The Triple Warmer Sound is an effective stress reducer. If done before going to sleep it helps you to get a good, deep, relaxing night's sleep.

The Triple Warmer does not have an emotion, Element or color associated with it. The Sound is H-E-E-E-E-E-E-E (pronounced with a long E).

1. Lie on your back (or recline in a chair) with your arms resting palms upward at your side.

2. Inhale fully as in this week's Regulating the Breath exercise, filling the lower abdomen, the middle chest and upper chest.

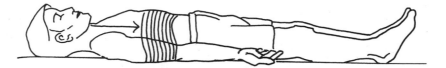

3. Begin to exhale as you subvocally make the Triple Warmer Healing Sound H-E-E-E-E-E-E-E.

4. Simultaneously flatten first your upper chest, then your middle chest region and finally your lower abdomen. Imagine that a large roller is moving down your body and squeezing out your breath, beginning at the top of your head and ending at the lower abdomen.

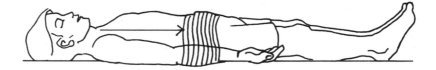

5. Rest and take a few normal breaths and imagine that all your major organs are relaxing.

6. Repeat at least 3 times per session.

This is the last of the Healing Sounds. Remember, you can do just the Healing Sound at any time; the movements make them even more effective.

You should continue doing the Healing Sounds every day. Begin with the Lung Sound and work your way to the Triple Warmer Sound. Do three of each. If you want to affect a single organ, just do that organ sound, but it is recommended that you try to do all of them every day.

Don't forget the Healing Sounds as we continue with the 100 Days of Practice. They are easy, efficient and effective.

Taoist Self-Massage Rejuvenation: The Neck and Throat

Air travels into and out of our body through our throat which lies inside the front part of our neck. The neck also contains the uppermost portion of our spinal column, the neck vertebrae. All the messages that pass downward from the head or up from the body must pass through the neck. As a result of this heavy traffic flow, our neck often becomes stiff, tight and painful. Negative emotions such as anger, fear, worry, depression and impatience all can cause stress and strain in the neck.

The Taoists referred to the throat as the Twelve Story Pagoda. It is highly susceptible to stress and strain. In many of us it is a source of constant nagging pain. The muscles in the throat often get weak as a result, losing mobility because of tight muscles on the back and sides of the neck.

In the middle of the throat are the thyroid and parathyroid glands. They also react to tension and stress. The Taoists believe that these two glands govern the powers of self-expression and courage. Tight neck muscles will constrict the throat. This can result in loss of mobility in the neck and loss of confidence and an inability to express yourself when speaking.

The throat is also a main thoroughfare for many of the body's energy meridians including both the Governor Channel up the back of the neck, and the Functional Channel down the front.

Releasing tension and stress from the neck and throat and keeping the neck soft and flexible will allow blocked energy to flow more freely and increase communication between your body and your brain. It will help you to speak better and feel more confident about yourself. Most important, you will feel better. Here are a number of exercises to relax, limber up and strengthen this most important part of your body.

Massaging under the Chin

1. Place your thumbs under the front of your chin.

2. Use your thumbs to press into and massage the muscles under the chin. Work your way back, on both sides, along the jawline, toward your neck. You might find some really sore spots along the way. Massage the sore spots. Go deep.

Very often you will find muscles that are so tense and painful that you cannot initially put a lot of pressure on them. If you massage every day, the pain and tightness should pass.

Massaging the Front of the Neck

1. Rub you hands together until hot.

2. Raise your right hand to your neck and spread the thumb apart, so that the front of your neck is between the index finger and the thumb.

3. Wipe down the neck from the chin to the bottom of the throat.

4. Alternate hands and wipe down with the left hand as above.

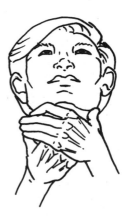

5. Continue alternating hands 9 to 36 times.

6. Massage the front of the throat including the thyroid and parathyroid glands, using the thumb and index, middle and ring fingers of one hand.

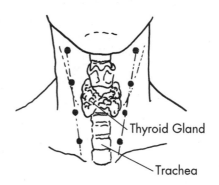

7. Using the 4 points in the diagram as a general guideline for the massage, find any painful points and massage them until they release.

Massaging the front of the neck and throat should help improve your powers of speech, increase your sense of courage and self-confidence, and improve your metabolic rate.

Massaging the Back of the Neck

The back of the neck is another area that is often chronically tight and tense in many of us. Massaging this area will help to relieve the tension and break up toxins that accumulate and cause pain and headaches.

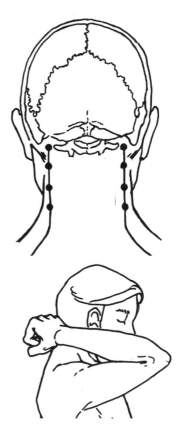

1. Make a fist with your right hand and use the base of the fist, on the pinkie finger side, or the knuckles to hit along the neck as shown in the diagram. Start at the bottom of the neck, where the shoulders and neck meet, and work your way up to the base of the neck.

2. Use the base or knuckles of your left fist to hit on the left side.

3. If you find any particularly painful or tense spots, massage them between your thumb and index, middle and ring fingers of either hand.

Crane Neck and Turtle Neck

These two neck stretching exercises were also among the first group of Taoist exercises that I ever learned. These two exercises mirror each other; each is the reverse of the other. Both work to compress and expand the spine as well as the disks and vertebrae of the neck. In both exercises the head and neck move in a circular motion. They can be done sitting or standing. I like to do these while I'm commuting to work in my car. The Crane Neck really opens up and loosens my throat and the Turtle Neck loosens up the back of my neck and upper shoulders. They are excellent warm-up exercises.

Crane Neck

1. Start with head and neck held straight.

2. Stretch your neck and head forward and upward.

3. When neck is fully extended, sink your chin down to the top of your chest.

4. Pull your head and neck back to the starting position. Repeat at least 3 times per session.

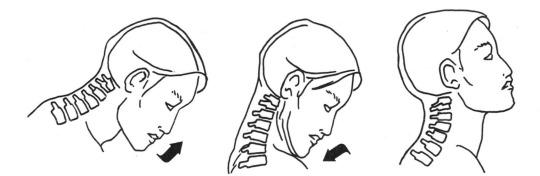

Turtle Neck

1. Start with head and neck held straight.

2. Sink your head down into your neck, like a turtle pulling its head into its shell, until your chin sits on top of your chest.

3. Push your chin outward from your body in a rising arc.

4. When your neck is fully extended, pull from the back of your head and neck until both are vertical and neck is somewhat stretched.

5. Repeat from step 2 above at least 3 times per session.

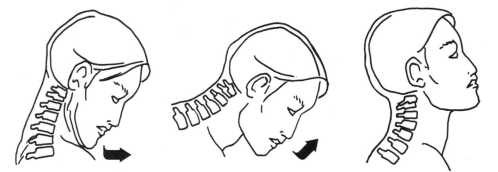

Yi Chin Ching: The Muscle-Tendon Change Classic—Part One

As we learned earlier in the story of Da Mo, the founder of Shaolin Kung Fu and Zen as well as Yi Chin Ching, it was also said that Da Mo meditated in a cave for nine years before he was ready to teach the Chinese Buddhist monks the exercises that formed the foundation of Shaolin Kung Fu.

Da Mo taught three different levels of exercise. Yi Chin Ching, the Muscle-Tendon Change Classic, comprises the first level. The primary aim of Yi Chin Ching is to strengthen the muscles and "grow" the tendons as you learn to direct Chi to your extremities.

The second and third levels are beyond the scope of this book. The second level is known as Bone Marrow Washing, which involves learning to absorb Chi directly into the fingertips and bones and the use of Sexual Energy to keep the bones strong and flexible. Advanced practitioners, both male and female, actually use weights as part of the training, tied either to the testicles or to a stone egg held in place inside the vagina. This practice was so secret that when I first learned it in 1983, my teacher, Mantak Chia, wouldn't even tell the group what we were about to learn until he was actually showing us what to do. (He did separate us into two groups, male and female, and his wife taught the women in another room. I understand that at later classes, the women "revolted" and refused to go to separate rooms. I guess you can't blame them. Taoist women are curious by nature.)

The third level is called Buddha Palm and consists of learning to transmit healing energy through the fingertips and palms by specific movements of the hands and fingers. These types of hand and finger movements are often called *mudras*.

These three levels of exercise formed the foundation of Buddhist martial arts, which in time were adopted by the Taoists into the practice known as Iron Shirt Chi Kung. Up until it was taught by Da Mo, the Chinese Buddhist monks were totally nonviolent. They meditated, they didn't exercise, and they certainly did not learn martial arts. Da Mo's teachings were quite controversial in his day and in the time after his death. But his teachings flourished at the Shaolin Temple. This was the birthplace of the type of Kung Fu that has, in more recent times, been memorialized in the television show of the same name.

In China today, there are numerous different sets of exercises that are called Yi Chin Ching. Some involve barely any movement at all, while some are fairly strenuous. Mantak Chia told me that he knows seventy different exercises that are called by this name. I know quite a few myself, but I obviously can't teach all of them. I do want to keep things simple. There are some underlying principles and movements that are necessary to know and understand in order to get the full benefit of Yi Chin Ching training. Many of the actual movements are even simpler than the Eight Pieces of Brocade. But there is a lot more going on than meets the eye, and I will do my absolute best to keep things clear and easy.

How to Stand: The Three Pumps

The Muscle-Tendon Change exercises are standing exercises although most can be adapted to a sitting position.

We do Abdominal Breathing with all the exercises. During the inhalation we relax. Upon exhalation we pull up on the perineum as we assume the proper posture. The perineum is considered to be the first pump.

The second pump is the Sacral Pump. The sacrum is the large triangular bone composed of five fused vertebrae in the lower portion of the spine that begins just above the coccyx (tailbone) and ends at approximately the level of the navel, at the point known as the Ming Men (Gate of Life). In most of us, the lower part of the sacrum tilts outward, away from the back, while the upper portion tilts inward toward the navel. If we straighten the sacrum, by tilting in the bottom, this acts as a pump to send Chi or Jing up the spine to the third pump.

The third pump is located at the back of the skull and is known as the Cranial Pump. This pump sends the Chi or Jing up to the top of the head. It is activated by pushing the head back and straightening the neck.

This is a very easy exercise to activate the three pumps:

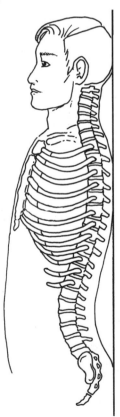

1. Stand up against a flat wall. Your feet can be either against the bottom of the wall or a few inches away, but your buttocks, upper back and the back of your head should be against the wall. Your arms are at your sides.

2. Do an Abdominal Breath inhalation, expanding the lower abdomen on all sides. Keep your body relaxed as you rest up against the wall.

3. Exhale and pull up on the entire perineum area, including the two front gates of the genitals, the perineum and the anus.

4. Pull in on the eye muscles and raise your tongue to the roof of your mouth.

5. Simultaneously tilt in your lower sacrum. You know you have accomplished this if there is no space between your lower back and the wall. In other words, flatten your lower back against the wall to activate the Sacral Pump.

6. You also push the back of your head against the wall so that the back of your neck is close to or flush against the wall and seems to stretch upward. To get a better feel for this, pull in your chin and use the tip of your right index finger to push your head back from the point directly under your nose (the Yen Chong point you learned about in Week One's Taoist Self-Massage Rejuvenation: Massaging the Lower Nose).

7. Inhale and relax. Do 6 times or more at each session this week.

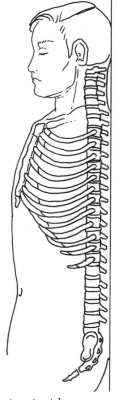

This is an important exercise for much of the future work. When your spine is flat against a wall, reach one hand behind you and try to push it between your lower back and the wall. If your hand squeezes through, you must increase the tilt of your lower sacrum toward your perineum.

Try pushing a hand through behind your neck. If there is space (and there probably will be) straighten your neck more. The muscles and tendons in the back of the neck can be in a lot of pain. The pulling in on the eyes is useful in reducing the strain and opening up blockages here. When you pull up on the perineum and in on the eyes you may feel something happening inside your spine. You may feel a tingle or a rush of energy up your spine. Activating the Three Pumps pushes spinal fluid up the backbone. Your Jing begins to rise. Perseverance is required.

Squeezing the Hands

Another important concept in Yi Chin Ching is squeezing or compressing the muscles. The idea is simple: upon exhalation, you just tighten and squeeze the muscles as if you were compressing them into your bones. It requires very little movement. We will begin by squeezing the muscles and tendons of the hands.

1. Hold both hands in front of you with palms facing each other, four to six inches apart. Your fingers are held open and apart. Your elbows are bent and face downward.

2. Inhale and keep hands and arms relaxed.

3. Exhale and squeeze the muscles of your fingers and hand into the bones. This requires very little movement. Your fingers go from soft to rigid as you exhale and squeeze. Don't squeeze the muscles of your forearm or upper arm; keep them soft (or try your best to keep them soft).

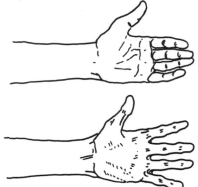

4. As you exhale and squeeze, mentally direct Chi down through your shoulders, arms and palms and into your fingertips.

5. Use your mind to momentarily feel the tip of each finger: both thumbs, both index fingers, both middle fingers, both ring fingers, and both pinkies. This is important!

6. Inhale and relax. Do at least three times per session. Try doing 3 or more sessions per day this week.

It may be difficult for you to squeeze just your hands without squeezing the rest of your arms as well. Since I'm not there to tell you if you're doing it right, I can only advise you on how to check yourself. Hold one arm limply in front of you, and use your other hand to feel how the muscles are soft when not flexed. If they are still flexed, this means that you are not relaxing these muscles and you must will them or command them to relax. The Yi Mind functions to direct your concentration to a specific location in your body; this in turn draws the Chi to this point, which in turn increases the flow of blood at and around the point of concentration.

If these muscles still don't relax and soften, just continue doing this exercise. Massaging the muscles of the arm might help. Having someone massage them for you might be even more helpful.

When you squeeze your fingers and hands the muscles of your forearms and upper arms should remain essentially soft, although you may feel some movement under the skin. It is easier to relax the upper arm than it is to relax the forearm. Practice until you get it.

The Inner Smile: The Middle Line

THIS WEEK WE ADD THE middle line to our practice of the Inner Smile. The middle line consists of our digestive system. I'm going to change the format for this week's practice, and give you a transcription of the middle line practice from a tape I recorded for myself some years ago.

Shen **Mind**

1. Repeat last week's lesson through step 12 completing the entire front line Inner Smile of the five major internal organs.

2. Become aware once more of the smiling energy in your eyes. Let it flow down to your mouth. Become aware of your tongue which is raised to the roof of your mouth. This connects the two major Channels of Energy, the Governor and the Functional Channels.

Bring the smiling Energy to the jaw, and feel the jaw releasing the tension that is commonly held there. Smile into your neck and throat, also common areas of tension. Although the neck is narrow, it is a major thoroughfare for most of the systems of the body. Air, food, blood, hormones and signals from the nervous system all travel up and down the neck. When you are stressed, the systems are overworked. The neck is jammed with activity and you get a stiff neck. Be like the Taoist Master and think of your neck as a turtle's neck and let it sink down into its shell. Let it rest from the burden of holding up your heavy head. Smile into your neck and feel the Energy opening your throat and melting away the tension.

Smile into the front part of your neck, where the thyroid and parathyroid glands are located. This is the seat of your power to speak and when it is stuck, Chi cannot flow. When it is tense and tight, you cannot express yourself. You will be frightened in front of a crowd, cowardly and your ability to communicate will break down. So smile down to the thyroid and parathyroid glands and feel your throat open like a flower blossoming.

Let the energy of the smile flow down to the thymus gland, the seat of rejuvenation and healing, loving energy. Smile down into it, feel it start to soften and moisten, feel it grow bigger like a bulb and gradually blossom. Feel the warm energy and healing Chi flow out of the thymus.

Return your attention to your tongue and make some saliva by working your mouth and swishing your tongue around. Put the tip of your tongue to the roof of your mouth. Tighten the neck muscles and swallow the saliva hard and quickly, making a gulping sound as you do.

With your inner smile follow the saliva down the esophagus and into the stomach, located at the bottom and below the left side of the rib cage. Thank it for its important work in liquefying and digesting food. Feel it grow calm and comfortable. Sometimes we abuse our stomach with improper food. Make a promise to your stomach that you will give it good food to digest. Smile into the small intestine, the duodenum, the jejunum and the ilium in the middle of the abdomen. It is about seven yards long in an adult. Thank it for absorbing food nutrients to keep you vital and healthy. Feel the smile travel through the small intestines.

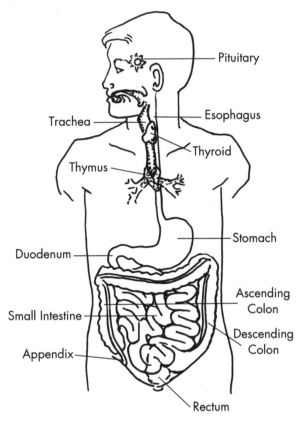

Smile into the large intestines. The ascending colon starts on the right side of the hip bone, and passes upward to the undersurface of the right lobe of the liver. The transverse colon passes downward from the right liver region across the abdomen to the left side, beneath the lower end of the spleen. The descending colon passes downward through the left side of the lumbar region and the sigmoid colon which lies within the pelvis. The large intestines end at the rectum and the anus. The large intestines are about a yard and one-half long. Thank them for eliminating wastes and for making you feel clean, fresh and open. Smile into them and feel them become warm, comfortable and calm. Return your concentration to your eyes and smile in your eyes.

3. Repeat last week's steps 13 through 20 to Warm the Stove and collect
   the energy in the Tan Tien.

THIS WEEK WE APPROACH THE halfway point in our training. By now you should be noticing some real changes
in your breathing habits. Abdominal Breathing should
be much easier for you to do. For some of you it may
have once again become your natural way of breathing.

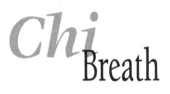

Chi Breath

If you are finding the pace I've set too demanding, slow down the pace.
Take two or three weeks to do a complete week's lesson. It is also important to
go back and review what you've learned. I have tried to design this book so
that what you learn each week generally builds on what you learned the week
before. So if you don't believe that you're ready to move on to the next week's
lessons, then take a week to review what you've learned. You could start back
at Week One and the next day do the Week Two exercises, then Week Three
and so on until you are ready to undertake the current week's exercises. This
is a good way to review and determine your progress. You might find that you
are bringing a whole new level of insight and understanding into your personal practice when you review.

A word of caution: don't jump around too much. If you do, you may soon
find that you've so scrambled up the system that you have ceased to make any
progress or feel confused about what you are doing. This is the point where
many students begin to lose interest and drop away from the practice. If this
should happen, if you find yourself drifting, then it is time for you to make a
firm determination to redouble your effort. Remember you are your own Master. You are not doing these exercises for my benefit. You are doing them to
take care of and nurture your greatest possession.

So take a moment to consider all you've learned up to now. Do you feel any healthier than when you began learning the 100 Days of Practice, or do you feel worse? Are you breathing better? Do you feel stronger or more flexible than when you began? Do you want to continue?

If you answered these questions in the affirmative, then you are ready to move on to Week Seven. For those of you who are still unsure, my advice is to stick with it. The best is yet to come.

Ming Men Breathing

For many weeks now I have been telling you that Perineum Power can be used to direct Chi to various points in the body. This week you will learn how to do this.

We have been using Perineum Power since Week Three. I'm sure that many of you have felt Energy rise upward through your body when you pulled up on the entire perineum area or on its various component parts: the sexual organs, the perineum or the anus. Up till now I have not given you specific instructions on how to control the Energy aside from telling you to pull up on the perineum.

The secret to controlling the flow of Chi is to push the proper part of the perineum toward the specific point you want it to travel to. A few weeks ago, this might have sounded impossible or nonsensical to you, but if you have been doing your exercises regularly, this should now make perfect sense.

This week we will learn to direct Energy to the Ming Men (Door of Life) point on the spine. This point is directly opposite the navel. It is easily located by placing your right pointer finger in your navel and your left thumb on your spine at the same level as the navel. If you bend forward from the waist, the vertebra opens here as you bend.

You will do an Abdominal Breath and expand the lower abdomen. Before exhaling you will pull in the navel toward the Ming Men and simultaneously pull up on the anus and mentally direct it, as if you were pushing it upward and backward toward the Ming Men. This is difficult to describe in words. Some of you will feel as if the anus is being pushed upward from below, while others might feel that it is being pulled upward from the Ming Men. This exercise makes use of the Yi mind to direct the flow of Chi. Version A is as follows:

1. Inhale slowly, expanding the lower abdomen and filling the lower, middle and upper parts of the lungs.

2. Hold your breath and pull in your navel toward your spine.

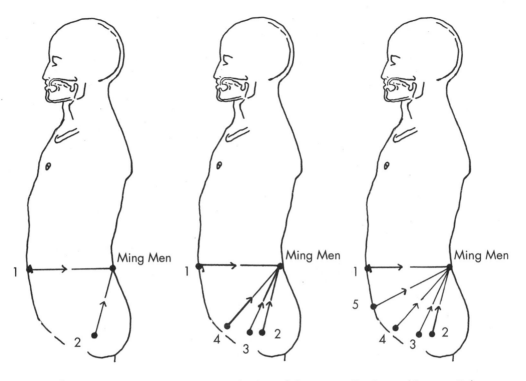

1 – Navel   2 – Anus   3 – Perineum   4 – Sexual Organs   5 – Sperm/Ovarian Palace

3. Simultaneously pull up on your entire anus, paying special attention to rear part on the coccyx side (tailbone) of the anus, and direct it upward and backward toward the Ming Men point on the spine directly opposite the navel.

4. Exhale slowly and contract the abdomen as you continue to pull up on the anus and direct it toward the Ming Men.

5. When fully exhaled, release the pull on the anus.

6. Begin another breath. Do at least 9 per set. Eighteen or more are recommended.

This exercise may be difficult for some at first. If so, try Version B, pulling the entire perineum area: sexual organs, perineum and anus toward the Ming Men. This variant is very powerful, so don't overdo it. Version C is an even more powerful version, pulling from the Sperm or Ovarian Palace just above the sexual organs on the Functional Channel. When you pull in on all of these areas and direct each and all of them toward the Door of Life, you might feel the Energy expand out from the spine and flood the entire kidney region on both sides of the body. Don't pull too strenuously. Start off very gently.

We will make further use of this exercise in this week's Yi Chin Ching lesson in the Regulating the Body section.

The Six Healing Sounds

You have now learned all six Healing Sounds. There are no more to teach you. But I don't want you to forget them. You can do a Healing Sound with almost all the exercises in the Regulating the Breath and Regulating the Body sections of this book. You can do them when you practice the Inner Smile. Do the proper sound as you smile into each of the five major organs. Do one of the Healing Sounds as you exhale. They also work wonders in relieving the stress and strain of negative emotions. They provide us with a tool to use to eradicate the negative and build up the positive. Use the Lung Sound when you are sad or depressed; the Kidney Sound when you are feeling fearful (I find this one particularly effective).

Recently I attended the annual International Healing Tao Instructors-Teachers Training session in the desert outside of Sedona, Arizona. One afternoon some of us took an unscheduled hike up a mountainside. I wasn't wearing the best shoes to do this and soon found myself unable to cross an open ledge to get to safer ground. My feet just wouldn't move. The only thing I could think of doing was the Kidney Healing Sound. As soon as I started doing it, I felt the heat escaping out of my kidneys and my body readjusting to the internal temperature change. Within a few seconds I was able to walk across the ledge.

The Liver Sound counters anger. The Heart Sound is good for a whole bunch of negativity: hatred, cruelty, hastiness, impatience. The Spleen Sound calms worry and anxiety.

You also have a whole set of seated Healing Sound Chi Kung in your repertoire of exercises. You can do them in the morning or evening or any time you have the opportunity.

Here is another simple form of Healing Sound Chi Kung that can be done virtually any time and any place. Just as the five major internal organs are linked to five external organs, such as the ears and nose and also to parts of the eyes, there is also a connection between the five fingers of the hands and the five major internal organs and Five Elements. The following chart details the correspondences:

HEALING SOUND	FINGER	ORGAN	ELEMENT	NEGATIVE EMOTION
WH-O-O-O-O	Thumb	Spleen/ Pancreas	Earth	Worry, Anxiety
S-S-S-S-S-S-S	Index Finger	Lungs	Metal	Sadness, Grief, Worry
H-A-W-W-W-W	Middle	Heart	Fire	Hatred, Cruelty, Impatience
SH-H-H-H-H-H	Ring Finger	Liver	Wood	Anger
CHU-W-A-A-Y	Pinkie Finger	Kidneys	Water	Fear

The way to do the exercise is to hold a finger from one hand, inside the fist of the other and gently twist and pull on the finger as you do the Healing Sound. It is also a good way to massage the fingers. It can be done standing or sitting.

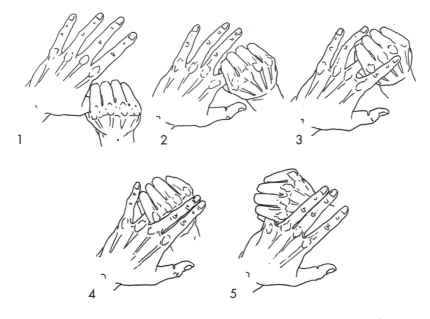

1 – Spleen/Pancreas   2 – Lungs   3 – Heart   4 – Liver   5 – Kidneys

Taoist Self-Massage Rejuvenation: Spinal Cord Breathing

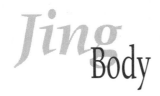

IF I ONLY HAD TIME to do one exercise, and I wanted to get my Chi flowing, this is probably the one I would do.

Spinal Cord Breathing is an excellent exercise that can be done either standing or sitting. It works to relax the spine and back muscles and activate the sacral and cranial pumps and the thymus and adrenal glands. The spine is the major pathway of the Governor Channel. The more relaxed the spine is, the more easily Energy can flow through it.

This is a fairly vigorous exercise.

1. Exhale and relax.

2. Inhale and tilt the lower sacrum back, away from the perineum. Simultaneously, push your head back toward your shoulders so that you are looking upward. This creates a large arch in the middle of your back.

3. Push your abdomen and chest outward, to expand your ribcage and activate the thymus and adrenal glands.

4. Make a fist with both hands and bring both fists up to shoulder level, bending both arms at the elbow. Pull back on the elbows and shoulders, as if trying to bring your scapulae (shoulder blades) together.

5. Press your neck into your shoulders to activate your cranial pump and clench your teeth.

6. Exhale and tilt the lower sacrum and head forward, rounding your back.

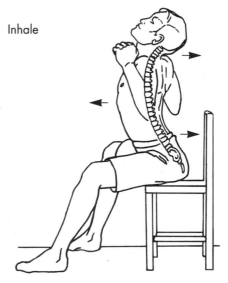

Inhale

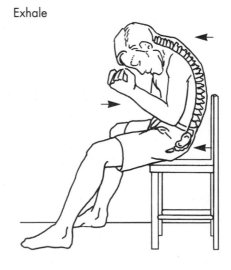

Exhale

7. Bring your elbows, forearms and fists forward in front of your body and together into the chest. Sink your rib cage and sink your chin into your upper chest. Do not tighten your muscles, just relax.

8. Repeat at least 9 times per session. If you do this exercise when standing, stand with feet facing forward, shoulder width apart.

Yi Chin Ching: The Muscle-Tendon Change Classic–Part Two

You have been learning Yi Chin Ching from the inside out. Rather than simply showing you the forms, you have been learning the details, which, when put all together, will allow you to get the maximum benefit from The Muscle-Tendon Change Classic. I can appreciate the difficulty in learning this from a book. There is no one there to correct you if you are doing it wrong. However, I also see the benefits of learning from a book. We can proceed slowly and methodically, step-by-step. This is not the way I first learned them. I learned the forms and not the details from a teacher who spoke broken English. It took years, with my teacher's improving command of the language, before I was able to understand all the details that make these exercises work. You are the beneficiary of my years of study and practice. The details are not difficult to follow if you carefully read the instructions and go step-by-step as we have been doing.

How to Stand–Part Two

What you are about to learn is easy for me to describe, but as a practical matter is one of the most difficult aspects of Chi Kung for Westerners to understand and accomplish.

For many of us, our shoulders are the tightest parts of our body. They are often the source of constant aches and pains that only seem to get worse as we age. Poor posture and improper alignment of the shoulders are generally the culprits.

Yi Chin Ching training aids to develop or reestablish the natural alignment of the shoulders. This is accomplished by widening the shoulder blades out to our sides and allowing them to drop down into place.

Proper alignment of our shoulders is necessary to equalize the space in the upper part of our torso. If our shoulders are rolled forward, this compresses the width of our chest and decreases our lung capacity. If our shoulders are pulled back this causes our upper back to contract, our shoulder blades become rigid and our upper spine is compressed. All of this can become quite painful in time.

When held properly as we stand against a wall, the shoulders are slightly dropped and rounded. To accomplish this:

1. Stand against a wall as you learned last week. Inhale and expand the lower abdomen.

2. Without exhaling, pull in your navel toward your spine and pull up on your anus and direct it toward the Ming Men as you learned in this week's Regulating the Breath exercise. This will help in pushing the middle of your back against the wall.

3. Exhale, maintaining the pull on the navel and anus, tilt in the lower sacrum to activate the sacral pump and push back your head to activate the cranial pump.

4. Push your shoulder blades flat against the wall, widening your shoulders so that the entire area of both shoulder blades is pushed against the wall.

5. With your arms hanging by your sides, round your shoulders by keeping the area between the two shoulder blades against the wall and dropping and slightly rolling the outsides of the shoulder blades forward, away from the wall.

6. Imagine that there is an egg held in place under each of your armpits. This helps you to widen, round and drop your shoulders. Feel the eggs there and round and drop your shoulders around them. Don't break them. Move the tips of your elbows outward, away from your sides. Your palms face backward.

7. Relax and inhale. Do 3 or more times per session.

Shoulder Widening Exercise

For those of you with misaligned, tight or painful shoulders here is an exercise that should help you to widen your shoulders out to your sides, rather than roll them forward or pull them back.

1. Stand against a wall. Do a Ming Men breath, exhale, hold the pull and activate the sacral and cranial pumps.

2. As you exhale, bend your elbows and hold them out to your sides as you bring both hands in front of you. Your right hand is held palm down above your left hand which is held palm up.

3. Grasp your right wrist with your left hand and grasp your left wrist with your right hand. The two grasped wrists are held at solar plexus level.

4. Try to pull your arms apart from the elbows while maintaining your grasp on the wrists.

5. Drop your shoulders as you pull and feel your shoulders widen and push into the wall.

6. Relax and inhale a Ming Men breath.

7. Exhale, holding the pull and activate the sacral and cranial pumps and reverse the grasp so that your left hand is palm down above the palm up right hand as you grasp your wrists and pull as above.

8. Release the grasp, step away from the wall and drop your arms to your sides. Feel your shoulders relax as you maintain the widened and dropped position.

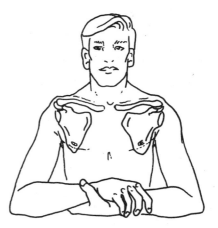

If your shoulders normally roll forward, when you do this exercise roll your shoulders back until the area between the shoulder blades is flush against the wall.

Squeezing the Feet

Just as you learned to squeeze your hands last week, this week you will learn to squeeze and compress your feet.

Our feet are the foundation of our entire stance. With our feet encased in often ill-fitting shoes, it is no surprise that many of us can't even distinguish the feel of our individual toes. They just feel like a mass of flesh down there. We lose sensitivity, muscles and tendons grow rigid and we lose mobility.

We want to direct Chi to our feet and activate them as we continue learning how to stand. Do this exercise barefoot or in socks.

1. Inhale and feel your feet in contact with the ground.

2. Exhale. Spread the toes out and squeeze the muscles of the toes.

3. Push and widen the balls of your feet into the ground. Squeeze the muscles. Feel as if you are clawing the ground with your feet. Don't squeeze the muscles of the calves and thighs.

4. Mentally direct Chi down your legs and into your feet.

5. Inhale and relax. Use your mind and try to distinguish the tip of each toe: the big toe, second toe, middle toe, fourth toe and pinkie toe of both feet.

6. Repeat 2 or 3 times per session.

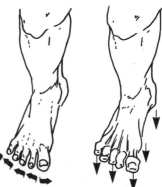

This exercise also functions to root us to the ground, a process we first learned in Week Three, Sexual Kung Fu for Men.

Next week we will learn to put all the Yi Chin Ching pieces together and begin doing the forms. Meanwhile continue to practice standing against a wall and Squeezing the Hands as you learned last week.

Sexual Kung Fu: Testicle and Ovarian Breathing–Part One

We are now reaching the core of Taoist Sexual Kung Fu. This involves learning how to bring the Sexual Energy (Jing Chi) up the spine and into the head to rejuvenate the brain.

I could probably teach all the steps of the process in this week's lesson, but you would never get the full results. So we are going to proceed slowly and methodically over the next five weeks. This way there is no reason you should not be able to raise your Jing. Don't be impatient. Don't jump ahead. These teachings are among the greatest gifts of the Taoists.

In China, you probably could not learn this. As I understand the current situation, the sexual practices have been suppressed along with the practices of internal alchemy. This is why I make a distinction between Chi Kung Masters in modern China and true Tao Masters. Recent books on Chi Kung (Qigong) practices coming out of mainland China barely mention sexuality at all. Their position on internal alchemy is summed up in *Qigong Essentials for Health Promotion*, by Jiao Guori (China Today Press, second edition, Beijing, China, 1990): "In ancient times Qigong was regarded as the key to immortality. This is impossible, because aging is an objective law. The purpose of undertaking Qigong is not to obtain immortality by closing the eyes and idling time away, but to build up physical stamina to avoid premature aging so that one can always be alert and vigorous and contribute more to mankind."

Actually, the sexual practices have been suppressed in China for almost a thousand years. Before that time the bedroom arts were considered to be a part of Traditional Chinese Medicine and flourished in a society that had no notion of Original Sin. After that time, highly conservative neo-Confucianists of the Sung and Southern Sung Dynasties (A.D. 960–1280) forbid the open discussion of sex, burnt the books and forced the practices to go behind closed doors or underground (they never completely disappeared especially among the Taoists). It is not that the neo-Confucianists were against sex. They were just against talking or writing about it. The Communists just continued along this line. However, a few of the ancient texts survived, often in the libraries of Japanese collectors. These ancient texts are still being discovered. The oral tradition never died, passed on by Tao Masters to their students. As these texts and a few surviving Tao Masters made their way to the West, these ancient practices once again came to light. They will now slowly become a part of Western sexuality, not because they are virtually unknown and no longer practiced in China, but because of their intrinsic value. Such is the nature of change. Old knowledge returns in a different time and a different place. The *I Ching* says that a movement is accomplished in six stages and the seventh brings return.

Part One of Testicle and Ovarian Breathing is rather different for men and women. After this week, the practice is pretty much the same for both sexes until we reach Part Five.

Testicle and Ovarian Breathing is concerned with activating and raising unaroused Sexual Energy. It is a key part of the practice of Single or Self-Cultivation and is very gentle and not forceful at all. It is not erotic, but rather a health, longevity and rejuvenation practice.

Testicle Breathing: Part One

This exercise can be done sitting, standing or lying down. The following instructions are for the sitting posture. Once you understand them, you can apply the same principles as you stand or lie down. Wear loose-fitting clothing, boxer shorts or wear nothing below the waist.

1. Sit up straight on the edge of a chair, with both feet on the floor. Your shoulders are slightly rounded and your chest relaxed. Your knees are shoulder width apart. Rest your hands palm down on your knees.

2. Your testicles should hang freely and unobstructed over the edge of the chair.

3. Put your concentration on the two testicles.

4. Breathe gently and raise the tip of your tongue to the roof of your mouth. You should be relaxed as you do this exercise.

5. Inhale slowly and without using any, or just the slightest, muscularity, try to pull up the two testicles. You can pull in lightly on your eyes, but do not use the muscles of the two front gates, the perineum or the anus to lift your testicles.

6. Use your mind and your breath to raise the testicles. Imagine that you are gently breathing down into your testicles, filling them with Chi and causing them to rise as you pull them up with your Yi mind.

7. Exhale slowly and lower the testicles. Repeat 9 times per set.

8. When you are finished, put your concentration on the space between the two testicles. You might feel cold energy spreading out through them.

The Sexual Energy you are activating here is cold Yin Energy. When you become sexually aroused, the Sexual Energy grows hot and Yang, and more forceful measures are needed to control it. To do this exercise properly you should be relaxed and not sexually aroused.

Sometimes when you do this exercise, the testicles seem to jump up and down in a comic manner, giving rise to another name for this practice—the Dance of the Testes. It might take a while before you get this exercise to work. That's why we're spending so much time on it. Most of you will probably not feel any cold Yin Energy for a while. When you do, it might be quite startling. I remember the first time I did, it was icy cold.

Ovarian Breathing: Part One

The most common meaning of Yin and Yang is woman and man. Woman is Yin and man is Yang. However, the Taoists recognized that within each of us there is both Yin and Yang Energy. A prime aim of Sexual Kung Fu is to balance the Yin and Yang in our body. That is why men activate Yin Energy in Testicle Breathing. The unaroused cold Yin Energy balances the normally hot Yang Energy of the male. For women, the opposite is true. In Ovarian Breathing warm Yang Energy is activated to balance the female Yin Energy.

These self-cultivation exercises allow the practitioner to find the Yin and Yang Energies within oneself alone. These exercises are not as well known as the Dual Cultivation practices which require the presence and participation of a member of the opposite sex. Dual Cultivation is the realm of sexual alchemy. I will discuss it in the final week of practice by which time you should be perfectly ready to deal with it. In the meantime I will reveal, as clearly and plainly as I can, the secret of activating and raising the unaroused Jing Chi up the back and into the brain. It is necessary to know this and practice it before you are ready to deal with raising aroused Sexual Energy to the brain. Aroused Sexual Energy is much more powerful than unaroused Jing Chi. At this point you are not ready to use it yet, but in a few weeks you will be. I'll tell you again: the best is yet to come.

Ovarian Breathing differs from Testicle Breathing because of the physical differences of the organs themselves, and the woman's menstrual cycle.

The Taoists found that during the menstrual cycle, the time between the end of the bleeding and ovulation is when the Essence of the ovaries is hottest or most Yang. This, then, is the time when the practice of Ovarian Breathing will be most beneficial, because you can actually draw Yang Jing Chi out of the egg. You can still practice at any other time during the cycle, including during menstruation. Regular practice should decrease the length of the bleeding cycle and thus preserve your Jing among the other benefits to be derived from the practice.

In Part One of Ovarian Breathing we will learn to bring Essence from the ovaries into the Ovarian Palace.

1. Sit up straight on the edge of a chair, with both feet on the floor. Your shoulders are slightly rounded and your chest relaxed. Your knees are shoulder width apart. Your tongue is raised to the roof of your mouth. Rub your hands together until hot.

2. Locate the Ovarian Palace by pointing both thumbs directly at each other over your navel and forming a triangle by touching the tips of both index fingers together. The point where the index fingers meet is the Ovarian Palace.

3. Keeping the triangle in place, slightly spread out the three other fingers of each hand against your body. Your ovaries lie beneath these fingers.

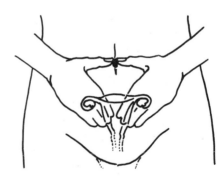

4. Place your concentration on your ovaries. Rub your fingers over your ovaries until you feel them begin to warm.

5. Use your Yi Mind to draw the warm Jing from the ovaries to the Ovarian Palace. (You may not feel heat right away. You might experience a tingling or swelling sensation. At this point as long as you feel something, that is sufficient.)

6. Simultaneously inhale a small sip of air and use your Yi Mind to very delicately close the lips of your vagina (like rose petals) to aid in drawing the Essence to the Ovarian Palace.

7. Exhale and open the lips of the vagina and relax. Repeat at least 9 times per session. Do a lot more if you have the time. Gently. Very gently.

The Inner Smile: The Back Line

Shen
Mind

ARE YOU SMILING YET? You've learned to smile into your eyes, into your major organs and into your entire digestive system. You've learned to connect your smiling eyes with the corners of your mouth. This week you will learn how to smile into the Back Line, which includes the brain, spine and the entire nervous system.

You have been learning the Inner Smile at a leisurely pace. This has allowed me to teach it to you in depth, step by step. By the end of this week's lesson, though, it may begin to seem a bit drawn out and unwieldy. What you should realize is that once you know the entire Inner Smile practice, it can be done rather quickly. You will have lots of opportunity to practice because all the remaining Regulating the Mind exercises are begun with the Inner Smile. You should get quite proficient at it and be able to do all three lines: front, middle and back in just a minute or two. This week though we are still learning, so we will still take it slow and methodically.

You also have been Warming the Stove in the Lower Tan Tien. This will be the fourth week. It may be that you have begun to feel some warmth in your lower abdomen after doing the Bellows Breathing. If you are, you might feel it move into other parts of your body as well. There's no telling where it might move to on its own. This is the body's own healing Energy. Only your body knows where it is needed.

I hope you have been Warming your Stove. It provides the foundation for the circulation of the Microcosmic Orbit which we will begin learning next week. If you are not feeling warmth, don't worry, just keep doing the exercise and continue with the 100 Days of Practice.

1. Begin by sitting up straight on a chair with both feet flat on the ground, legs together and hands clasped in your lap. The tip of your tongue is raised to the roof of your mouth.

2. Put your awareness on the tip of your nose, move up to the bump on the nose and then to the Third Eye.

3. Imagine a smiling Sun (don't use the Moon for this exercise) smiling right into your eyes. Smile into the outer and inner corners of both eyes, into the pupils, irises, whites and upper and lower lids, and feel the connection to the corners of your lips.

4. Do the Front Line Smile into the five major organs.

5. Swallow saliva and do the Middle Line Smile into the neck, stomach, large and small intestines, colon and anus.

6. Collect the power of the smile in the Third Eye. With your inner eyesight direct your smile 3 inches straight back into the Pituitary Gland. Feel the gland open up and blossom. Feel the smiling energy around the Pituitary Gland expand, encompassing the entire Crystal Palace which includes the Thalamus and Pineal Gland. This is the power center of the nervous system. Feel the center of your brain expand with bright golden light shining throughout your brain.

7. Move your smile like a great shining light up to the left side of the brain. Move the inner smiling eyesight back and forth throughout the left hemisphere of the brain. Move it up and down, back and forth, until you have filled the entire left side of your brain with radiant smiling energy.

8. Now move the Inner Smile across to the right brain. Move it up and down and back and forth in the right hemisphere until you have filled the right brain with radiant smiling, loving energy.

9. Bring the golden radiating smile to the front of your brain and move it straight back through the middle of the brain. The boundary between the left and right brain dissolves. The smile then turns downward to the cerebellum at the base of the skull. Smile into the cerebellum. This will balance the left and right brain and strengthen your nerves.

10. Move the Inner Smile down to the mid-brain, where the brain meets the upper-most vertebrae of the neck. Feel it expand and soften and enter the spinal cord. Starting at the cervical vertebrae at the base of the skull, move the Inner Smile. Bring this loving radiating energy down inside each vertebra and the disk below it. Count out each vertebra as you smile down through your spine. Move down through the seven cervical vertebrae of the neck, one by one.

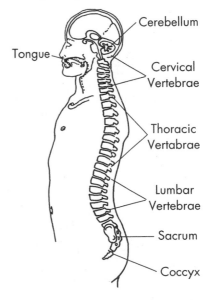

Cerebellum

Tongue

Cervical Vertebrae

Thoracic Vertabrae

Lumbar Vertebrae

Sacrum

Coccyx

11. When you finish the vertebrae of the neck, you continue into the twelve thoracic vertebrae behind the chest, one by one.

12. Next smile into the five lumbar vertebrae of the lower back, one by one.

13. Continue into the sacrum, smiling into the triangular bone composed of five fused vertebrae.

14. Finally smile into your coccyx, the tailbone at the very tip of your spine.

15. Your entire spine is now filled with smiling golden radiating light. Feel your spinal cord and back become loose and comfortable. Feel the disks softening as you smile into them. Feel your spine expanding and elongating, making you feel taller. The smiling radiant energy fills your entire spine and moves out from your spine into all the nerves of your body.

16. Feel the Inner Smile radiate outward into your arms and hands. Smile into your fingers, feel the tips of each finger smiling and glowing like a tiny sun.

17. Smile downward into your sexual organs and then your legs, through your knees and calves and into your feet. Smile into your toes and feel the tips of all your toes smiling and shining like tiny suns. Feel your whole body smiling and radiating golden light.

18. Return your Inner Smile to the Third Eye area. Use your tongue to create saliva and smile golden radiating light into the saliva. Swallow the saliva and follow its path down to the Lower Tan Tien. Do Bellows Breathing to Warm the Stove. Do at least 18 rapid breaths.

To close:

19. *Men:* Spiral energy clockwise around the navel 36 times then reverse counter-clockwise 24 times. *Women:* Spiral counter-clockwise around the navel 36 times then clockwise 24 times.

20. Rub your palms together until hot and massage your face. Rub them again and cover the eyes and absorb the Chi into your eyes.

21. *Men:* Place your left palm over your navel and cover it with your right palm. *Women:* Place your right palm over your navel and cover it with your left palm. Sit quietly like this for a minute or so to complete the exercise.

Your whole body should feel relaxed. The Back Line exercise increases the flow of spinal fluid and sedates the nervous system. Smiling into a disk keeps it from hardening and becoming deformed so it cannot properly absorb the weight of the body. Back pains can be prevented, eliminated and relieved by smiling into the spine.

week eight

WE NOW ENTER THE SECOND half of the training. This week we turn our attention to the Microcosmic Orbit. We are now at the heart of the practice.

Completion of the Microcosmic Orbit is the primary aim of this book. It is the secret of the Golden Flower. But the Golden Flower has many secrets. Last week you encountered another one of them. That was the light of the Crystal Palace that radiated throughout the brain and spine and finally into your whole body. That radiating light is the Golden Flower. I hope some of you experienced it. There is no doubt that the living presence of a Tao Master would increase the likelihood of such an experience. But, if you are properly relaxed and in the right frame of mind (that is, No Mind), then you might have experienced the golden light. If you didn't, in time you will.

Tan Tien Breathing

LAST WEEK YOU LEARNED THE powerful breathing technique called Ming Men Breathing in which you used Perineum Power to direct Chi to the point on the spine opposite the navel. This week I will teach you to use Perineum Power to direct Chi to the navel itself.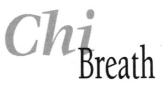

By doing this you are not only learning to direct the flow of Chi, but also to increase the internal pressure inside of your body. This concept of increasing Chi pressure will become more and more important as you work your way through the second half of the 100 Days of Practice.

Tan Tien Breathing is essentially a more powerful Abdominal Breath. It is an excellent exercise for strengthening the lower abdomen.

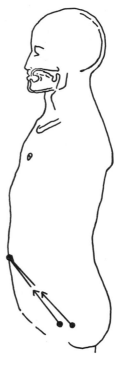

1. Do an Abdominal Breath, expanding the lower abdomen. Do not fill the middle or upper lungs with air.

2. Pause for a second and actually push your abdominal muscles forward so that they visibly expand around the navel, pushing your navel forward.

3. Simultaneously push your perineum and front part of the anus upward toward your navel.

4. Exhale and hold the pull.

5. Relax your abdomen, then inhale. Repeat at least 9 times per session.

In this week's Yi Chin Ching section we will combine this breath with Ming Men Breathing to create an even more powerful breathing technique.

Taoist Self-Massage Rejuvenation

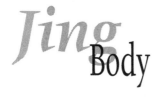

SOMETIMES WHEN I GET UP in the morning I'm just in no mood to do any exercise. I don't even want to think about exercising. Screwing the Hips is designed for mornings like this. It is a very simple movement that essentially consists of rotating the hips to the left in a circular motion and then rotating them to the right in a circular motion, activating the Sacral Pump as you move the hips forward and releasing the sacrum as you move the hips backward.

Screwing the Hips

This is also an excellent exercise for developing the muscles involved in sexual intercourse. It helps to develop the muscular control needed for extended sexual sessions.

1. Stand up with feet facing forward. They can be a few inches to shoulder width apart. Experiment and see what position is most comfortable for you.

2. Push your hips back so that your back arches a little, and your buttocks stick out.

3. Slowly move your hips to the left side.

4. Activate the Sacral Pump and rotate the hips forward on the left side.

5. Circle the hips to the right side then push the hips and buttocks backward and release the Sacral Pump.

6. Circle hips to the left and repeat above steps at least 3 times.

7. Repeat the exercise 3 times to right side, moving the hips forward and activating the Sacral Pump on the right side and releasing and moving the hips back on the left side.

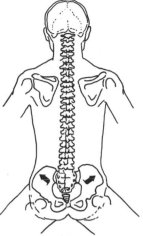

You can also try doing the exercise while seated. It helps relieve stress and tension when you sit too long. If you are in a crowded environment, just do small circles with the hips so as not to be too obvious.

The sexual implications of the exercise should be obvious. Mantak Chia was fond of saying that when you do this exercise with a partner, "you are really screwing." It allows for interesting angles of attack, as well as assorted long and short thrusts of the hips and genitals.

Hitting the Sacrum

This exercise is similar to other hitting exercises you have learned in this book, except this time you hit the sacrum. It is useful in loosening up the sacrum and sacral pump and in relieving sciatic pain which originates in the sacrum and shoots down the legs.

1. Rub your hands together until hot.

2. Contract the back of your anus toward the sacrum, directing Chi to the sacrum.

3. Make a fist with both hands.

4. Using the knuckle side of the fists, alternately hit both sides of the sacrum. Start at the top of the sacrum and work your way down to just above the coccyx.

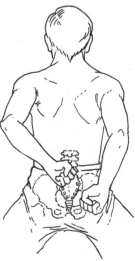

Yi Chin Ching: The Muscle-Tendon Change Classic—Part Three

Part of the real beauty of the Taoist practices is the way different parts of the system neatly fit together and interlock or lay the foundation for other parts of the practice. This is how I have constructed this book: interweaving exercises for regulation of the breath, mind and body to form one whole, coherent system.

The Muscle-Tendon Change Classic is in itself an entire system. Done properly, it regulates all Three Treasures: Chi, Jing, and Shen—Breath, Body, and Mind. When I first considered including Yi Chin Ching in this book, I felt as if I was faced with a truly daunting task. The various exercise forms are ridiculously easy. Each form involves just a single movement of the arms and hands which distinguishes it from the other forms. But I realized that if I just taught the forms, it would not be possible for you, the reader, to really get many results from the exercises.

You can see from the last two weeks that there are a lot of pieces that must fit together to get the Muscle-Tendon Change exercises to work. Very little has been written that provides a guide to the Western reader and practitioner on how to put together and coordinate all the various aspects of Muscle-Tendon Change Chi Kung into a practical and useful system. They are wonderful exercises that have been around for almost fifteen hundred years. I would like to review with you some of the many aspects of training that you have learned to show you how they do fit together.

First of all we have breathing. We have yet to learn the technique we will actually use with the Yi Chin Ching forms. But you have learned its various parts. You will combine Tan Tien Breathing, which you learned earlier this week in the Regulating the Breath section, with Ming Men Breathing. This is how it is done:

1. Inhale slowly and expand the lower abdomen.

2. Push out your navel and pull up your perineum and anus toward the expanded navel.

3. Without exhaling, pull your navel toward your spine and push your anus toward the Ming Men point on the spine.

4. Exhale slowly as you hold the pull.

5. Release and begin again.

For a more powerful pull you can also add the pull in on the Sperm or Ovarian Palace, sexual organs and perineum in step 3 above. First push out the navel then pull it back toward the Ming Men. Then pull up on the anus. As you begin to exhale pull in the Sperm or Ovarian Palace first, then quickly add first the sexual organs and next, the perineum. If you comprehend this, then you should pause a moment and realize how much you have learned. Surely what's mentioned above would have baffled or disgusted you before you read this book. But now I hope it makes perfect sense.

With this breathing technique you are also sending Chi to the two kidneys, which lie on either side of the spine. If you put your concentration there, you can feel the kidney region, on both sides, actually expand as you pull the navel and push up the anus toward the Ming Men. We are building a Chi Belt around the body at the level of the navel.

You have been doing a lot of strange exercises below the belt. A primary aim of Chi Kung is to strengthen the entire lower abdominal region including the sexual organs and the organs of digestion and excretion. If you have been doing the exercises in this book, you should be finding that not only is your lower abdomen in much better shape than before you began the practice, but you are now aware of and in conscious control of various parts of your lower anatomy that you had never before even considered. You should easily be able to distinguish between the perineum, anus and the sexual organs. This growing ability will serve you well as we continue with the 100 Days of Practice.

You have learned how to activate the Three Pumps: the Perineum Pump, the Sacral Pump and the Cranial Pump. This is crucial to strengthen the body, open the spine, send Sexual Energy up to the head and complete the Microcosmic Orbit.

You have learned how to stand and open the shoulders. This allows us to release tension in the scapula or shoulder blades. Dropping and rounding the shoulders actually stretches the muscles and tendons of the scapula. There is tremendous strength in the scapula. Taoist martial artists know that using the scapula to move the arm, rather than the muscles of the arm, allows for a strike that barely seems to move more than a few inches, but is devastatingly powerful. As we do the forms, I will show how to connect your scapula with the movement of your arms. This is a difficult technique to learn from a book, but I will at least teach you the rudiments of Scapula Power.

You've learned to squeeze your hands and feet. This compresses Chi into the muscles, tendons and bones. You also use your mind to direct the Chi into your hands and feet. All of these pieces work together in the Muscle-Tendon Change forms.

The forms you'll learn this week are somewhat modified and simplified from the original Chinese forms. You should find them easy and effective.

Forms 1–4

1. Stand up (it could be against a wall) with your arms raised in front of you and your hands at approximately shoulder height. Both hands are open and the palms face upward toward the sky. Your elbows are slightly sunk so that although your arms are in front of you, they are not quite straight.

2. Inhale and expand the lower abdomen. Pause and push your navel out and push your anus toward the navel.

3. Without exhaling, pull in your navel toward your spine and pull up on your anus and direct it toward the Ming Men and kidneys.

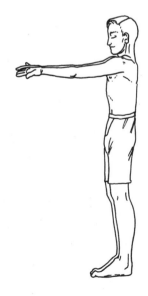

4. Exhale, maintaining the pull on the navel and anus, tilt in the lower sacrum to activate the sacral pump. Pull your chin in and push the base of your skull back to activate the cranial pump.

5. Round your shoulders and drop and roll your shoulder blades slightly forward.

6. Simultaneously squeeze your hands and straighten your elbows as your arms push forward from the scapula.

7. Also simultaneously squeeze your feet into the ground and then also squeeze your calves and thighs.

8. From your Tan Tien direct Chi to your hands and fingertips. Hold this position for a second or two.

9. Relax, sink the elbows and pull back the shoulder blades.

10. Inhale and repeat. Do 3 or more times per session. Shake your hands and then feet for a few seconds to end each session.

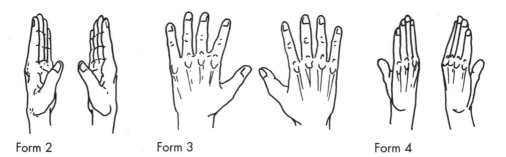

Form 2   Form 3   Form 4

Forms 2–4 are performed exactly the same way except in Form 2 the palms face each other. In Form 3 the palms face downward and in Form 4 the palms face outward, away from each other (the back of the palms face each other).

Practice these four forms this week. Next week you'll learn some more. But now you have the basic practice. Work on it until you find that you are establishing a rhythm, with your spine undulating back and forth as you activate and release the Sacral and Cranial Pumps.

I hope I have clarified the concept of Scapula Power. When you exhale, round the shoulders, flatten the upper back and push the shoulder blades slightly forward to move your arms. When you squeeze your hands, straighten the elbows. It is all right to squeeze the forearms and upper arms as well. You previously had learned how to isolate the hands and the feet while squeezing so you could learn how to direct Chi to the extremities. When you relax, sink the elbows in front of you and draw back the shoulder blades.

When done properly, these exercises have a rhythmical feel to them. I think they're a lot of fun.

Sexual Kung Fu: Testicle and Ovarian Breathing–Part Two

The aim of this week's lesson is the same for both men and women: to draw the Jing Chi to the perineum, the body's Sexual Energy collection point. Again, because of the anatomical differences, I will describe the exercises separately for each sex.

Testicle Breathing: Part Two

1. Begin by doing the Testicle Breathing you learned last week. You should be totally relaxed as you practice. After a few minutes you should feel cold energy. If you don't experience this—and many of you won't initially—just try to sense some energy or tingling feeling in your testicles.

2. Direct your mind to the perineum. Imagine that there is a silver straw running from your testicles up to your perineum.

3. Keep your point of concentration on the perineum and as you pull up the testicles, imagine that the cold energy flows into the silver straw and up to the perineum.

4. Inhale and draw the Jing Chi to the perineum.

5. When you exhale you keep your mind focused on the perineum to hold the Sexual Energy there. If you don't maintain this focus on the perineum, the Jing Chi will sink back to the testicles.

6. Repeat 9 times per session.

The concept here of using an imaginary silver straw to draw up the Jing Chi might need some explanation. When you were a kid and you sucked some liquid into a straw, if you placed a fingertip on the top of the straw, the liquid would not leak out the bottom. If you removed your finger, it would. Essentially we are doing the same thing here. We are using our Yi Mind to lead the Chi to the perineum and—just like the fingertip placed over the top of the straw—we keep our mind concentrated at the perineum, on the tip of the imaginary silver straw, and keep the Jing Chi from leaking away.

Ovarian Breathing: Part Two

1. Begin doing the Ovarian Breathing you learned last week.

2. Inhale a small sip of air and gently contract the lips of the vagina toward the perineum.

3. Gently contract and pull up on the perineum.

4. Imagine that there is a silver straw connecting your ovaries with your perineum. Use your mind to guide the warm Sexual Energy from your Ovarian Palace through the silver straw to the perineum.

5. Maintain your point of concentration at the perineum. This acts to "seal" the straw, to keep the Jing Chi from leaking away.

6. Pause for a moment and hold your breath and feel the flow of energy from the Ovarian Palace, to the vagina, clitoris and perineum.

7. Exhale and maintain your point of concentration on the tip of the imaginary silver straw.

8. Repeat 9 times per session.

The silver straw concept described above applies equally to men and women. As you practice, it will become easier for you to "hold" the Jing

Chi in place with your Yi Mind while continuing to use your mind to draw additional Jing Chi from the ovaries. Men too will find that they can maintain a "mental finger" on the silver straw while continuing to draw Sexual Energy from the testicles. This ability increases in importance in future weeks as we learn to draw the Jing Chi up the spine.

The Microcosmic Orbit: Part One

THERE ARE MANY WAYS TO learn the opening of the Microcosmic Orbit. As you should be aware by now, the Microcosmic Orbit consists of a linking of the Governor Channel which runs up the back with the Functional Channel which runs down the front of the body.

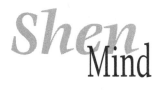

Opening the Microcosmic Orbit involves clearing all the obstructions that impede the flow of Chi through the Governor and Functional Channels. The Governor Channel is Yang, positive, and the Functional Channel is Yin, negative. When the Two Channels are joined by raising the tip of the tongue to the upper palate, they form a circuit called the Microcosmic Orbit or Small Heavenly Cycle. This allows a greater amount of Chi to circulate in the body and results in improved blood circulation and a balancing and strengthening of the Three Treasures: Energy, Essence, and Spirit (breath, body, and mind).

The Taoists believed that many systems of yoga and meditation, especially Kundalini Yoga, were dangerous in that they sought to raise large amounts of energy to the head. They found that overloading and overheating the head could result in headaches, delusions, mental imbalance and an inability to work or function in society. This is another reason the Microcosmic Orbit is so important. Energy is raised up to the head in the Governor Channel, but it is then lowered down the body in the Functional Channel. At the end of a session, the Energy is collected and stored in the Tan Tien behind and slightly below the navel, which is the body's prime storehouse for Chi, often called the Sea of Chi. Chi is not permitted to remain scattered throughout the body or in the head, it must always be collected, as you've learned, at the end of each Regulation of the Mind exercise.

You have already learned many of the points along the route of the Microcosmic Orbit. Some of you may have already experimented with circulating Chi in the Microcosmic Orbit. A few of you might have already experienced an opening of the Orbit. Sometimes it just opens spontaneously. Even if this has occurred there is always more to learn about the Microcosmic Orbit, so please continue with the lessons.

For most of you, the Microcosmic Orbit has yet to be completed. You will learn it slowly, step by step, so that by the end of the 100 Days of Practice everyone who has read this book and practiced regularly should be able to complete the Microcosmic Orbit. Once you have completed this book, the exercises you have learned, the sexual practices and the Microcosmic Orbit are yours for the rest of your life. You will be the owner of these wonderful tools that protect, rejuvenate, and lengthen the years you have to enjoy your Greatest Possession.

It is generally taught that the Microcosmic Orbit begins at the navel. For many weeks now you have been practicing Warming the Stove. The Stove is the location of the Navel Point also called the Tan Tien. It is generally found one and one-half to three inches inside the body and an inch to an inch and one-half below the navel. The exact location differs in all of us. If you have been experiencing warmth in the lower abdomen when you Warm the Stove, then this is the place to begin.

This week we will connect the Tan Tien with the Sperm Palace in men and the Ovarian Palace in women. You are all familiar with the location of these points. Both of them are on the Functional Channel.

1. From a seated position, focus on a point in front of you and then after a few moments lower your eyelids and shift your attention to the tip of your nose. As soon as you feel comfortable and focused on the tip, move your point of concentration to the "bump" on your nose and then up to the Third Eye area between the eyebrows.

2. Smile into both eyes and feel the connection between the corners of your lips and the outer corner of the eyes. (If you wish, you can activate the inner and outer corners of the eyes, the pupils, irises, whites and upper and lower lids and feel the connection to the corners of the lips.)

3. Do the front line smile, quickly smiling into the five major organs: the heart, lungs, liver, kidneys and spleen/pancreas. (The middle and back lines of the Inner Smile are optional according to the time you have available, but it is recommended that you do them a few times every week, especially the back line. The more you practice, the faster and easier it will be for you to do them.)

4. Close your eyes and smile into the Third Eye area. Reverse the smile back into your head behind the Third Eye Point. See or visualize this region glowing with golden light. (Hint: Try visualizing the tip of a burning Fourth of July sparkler.)

5. Circle your tongue between the outside of your teeth and the back of your lips 9 times. Place your tongue behind the teeth and circle in the

opposite direction 6 times. From the Third Eye Point, smile into the saliva that fills your mouth. Visualize or imagine that your saliva begins to glow with the golden light.

6. Place the tip of your tongue to the roof of your mouth just behind your teeth. Pull in your chin to activate the cranial pump and swallow the saliva with a gulping sound.

7. Visualize the golden light descending to your Tan Tien. As it descends, the Energy Centers in your throat, in the center of your chest and in your solar plexus begin to glow as the golden, smiling light passes through them.

8. Place your attention on the Tan Tien. Look down with your inner eyesight.

   Do at least 18 Bellows Breaths (rapid Abdominal Breathing) to Warm the Stove.

9. Listen down to the Tan Tien. Hear your breathing slow down and become silent as you switch to Slow Fire (long, even Abdominal Breaths). Do this for a couple of minutes.

10. Inhale with your concentration on the Tan Tien and exhale and drop your concentration to the Sperm or Ovarian Palace.

11. Concentrate on the Sperm or Ovarian Palace. To do this properly, use your Yi Mind to shift your concentration to the Sperm or Ovarian Palace, use your inner eyesight to see or visualize it and listen down with inner hearing to maintain silent breathing. Do this for 2 or 3 minutes. The area might become warm.

12. Inhale and raise your concentration back to the Tan Tien. The Chi or warm current will follow, rising up from the Sperm or Ovarian Palace.

13. Exhale and move your concentration back to the Sperm or Ovarian Palace, and feel the Chi or a warm current follow from the Tan Tien. Go up and down 9 times, up on the inhalation and down on the exhalation.

14. Return your concentration to the Tan Tien and collect the energy.

   Men: Put your left hand over your navel and cover it with your right hand. Use your mind to circle the navel, in 3-inch circles, 36 times clockwise (from above down on the left side and come up on the right side) and then reverse 24 times counter-clockwise. On the final circulation draw the Chi into the Lower Tan Tien.

   Women: Put your right hand over your navel and cover it with your left hand. Use your mind to circle the navel, in 3-inch circles, 36 times counter-clockwise (from above down on the right side and come up on the left side) and then reverse 24 times clockwise. On the final circulation draw the Chi into the Lower Tan Tien.

Both Men and Women: Rub your palms together until warm and Massage your Face. Rub them again and cover the eyes and absorb the Chi into your eyes.

Reverse Breathing

REVERSE BREATHING IS THE SECOND of the two main breathing techniques of the Taoists. It is sometimes referred to as Taoist Breathing because it was a uniquely Taoist Chi Kung technique while Abdominal Breathing was supposedly a Buddhist Chi Kung technique adopted by the Taoists. Throughout the centuries the Taoists absorbed many Buddhist practices and made them their own. In many Chinese sources I have examined, it is virtually impossible to separate the Taoist aspects from the Buddhist, they are so interwoven. The Taoists' prime concern was "does it work?" rather than where it came from. The same holds true today. I have often seen experienced Taoists instantly change some facet of training or practice they have been working on for years when presented with a better or improved technique. Flexibility is a key to understanding the Taoist mindset.

Reverse Breathing is the reverse of Abdominal Breathing. On inhalation, the lower abdomen is pulled in toward the spine and upon exhalation it is released to expand to normal size. There is a natural inclination to tighten and pull up the diaphragm when you first begin practicing Reverse Breathing. That is why I have waited until the second half of the 100 Days of Practice to teach it to you.

The Abdominal Breathing that you have been practicing since Week Two should have made you conscious of your diaphragm and your ability to control it. It is important to keep the chest relaxed and to push down the diaphragm as you do Reverse Breathing. If you don't push the diaphragm down, your upper body will tense up and your heartbeat will increase. This is not what you want to have happen. Practice with attention to this detail.

Reverse Breathing has all the health benefits of Abdominal Breathing. It massages and strengthens the lower abdomen. It allows for a greater ability to direct Chi to the extremities and complete the Microcosmic Orbit. It also lays the foundation for Compression Breathing (a sexual practice) and Packing Process Breathing that you will learn later in the practice.

Another name for Reverse Breathing is Prenatal Breathing. Herein lies the secret of this breathing technique. The one aim of Chi Kung is to restore the Prenatal Chi that circulated in your body before you were born and much of the process is involved with rejuvenating the body. Abdominal Breathing re-creates the way we breathed as infants and young children. Reverse Breathing re-creates the way we breathed while we were still inside our mother's womb before we were born. This is the way a fetus breathes. This is the way you will now learn to breathe. It is a powerful, invigorating breath.

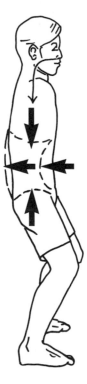

1. Begin by doing 3 Abdominal Breaths. At the final exhalation pull in your lower abdomen and flatten your stomach.

2. Inhale slowly and pull the lower abdomen toward your spine. As you do this, you will feel a downward pressure on your perineum.

3. Pull up on your perineum and sexual organs and simultaneously push down and lower your diaphragm.

4. Exhale and release the sexual organs and diaphragm. Imagine that you are exhaling right through the walls of the lower abdomen which expands on all sides.

5. Do at least 6 Reverse Breaths at each session.

Lowering the diaphragm is the hardest part of Reverse Breathing. Try smiling into the diaphragm to help it to relax. With practice you should be able to raise or lower your diaphragm at will, using your Yi Mind to control it.

Reverse Breathing doesn't replace Abdominal Breathing; it supplements it. We will make use of both techniques as we continue with the 100 Days of Practice.

Taoist Self-Massage Rejuvenation: Abdominal Massage

IN THE WEST, ABDOMINAL MASSAGE is almost unknown. Among the Taoists, it was developed to a fine art. Abdominal Massage is vital to cleaning toxins out of our body. When you wake up in the morning in a foul mood, depressed, sluggish or achy, this is generally the result of too many toxins in your system.

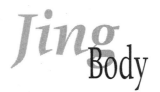

Abdominal Massage also helps the digestive process and relieves constipation by releasing knots and blockages. It also softens hard and enlarged lymph nodes in the navel area and can help to cure numerous illnesses.

The theory here is part of traditional Chinese medicine and is totally alien to Western medicine. The Chinese believed that gases and air trapped in the body are the cause of a whole host of ailments and problems. Chinese doctors call these *Sick Winds*.

Not all wind in the body is sick. The breathing process moves air in and out of the body. Air is wind. Gases are also formed in our bodies by the foods that we eat and the beverages we drink. A toxic environment, changes in the weather or the season, tension and negative emotions can all result in the accumulation of gases or wind in our bodies. It is only when this air or gas becomes trapped in our body and organs that it becomes Sick Wind. Abdominal Massage is vital to clearing out and releasing the Sick Winds.

Sick Winds cause blockages and knots in our body that result in the accumulation of toxins. Our lymph system functions to clear these toxins, but when the winds become stagnant and toxins build up the lymph nodes around our navel (as well as those under our armpits and in our neck) become hard, swollen and painful. Abdominal Massage helps to release the toxins and relieve the pain, stiffness and swelling of the lymph nodes.

As I mentioned, the Taoists developed Abdominal Massage to a healing art form. I will give you a basic but effective method to release the Sick Winds.

We will massage around (not on) the navel. You might be surprised to find that there is a great deal of tightness and pain around the navel. The area around the navel will be divided into eight separate sections, and we will massage each of these eight areas in a particular pattern. This technique is a simplification of a method known as Opening the Wind Gates.

You can use your thumb or bring the back of both palms together and use the index, middle and ring fingers of each hand to message each of the eight areas. Move the thumb or fingers in a circular motion applying as much pressure as you can take in each area. If the area is extremely painful, start off very gently.

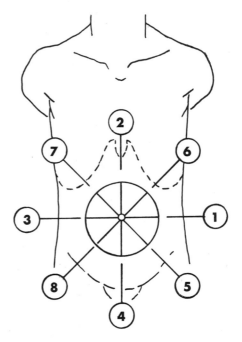

1. Begin on the left side of the navel, about an inch away from the navel. Massage here for 10 to 20 seconds, moving toward the left side of the body. Spend extra time massaging if the area is tight or knotted. Massaging here will also affect the Wind in the left kidney.

2. The second area is directly above the navel. Massaging here will affect the Wind of the heart.

3. The third area is on the right side of the navel. Massaging here affects the Wind of the right kidney.

4. The fourth area is below the navel. Massaging here affects the Wind of the sexual organs and bladder.

5. The fifth area is on the left side between the fourth and first area. Massaging here affects the Wind of the intestines.

6. The sixth area is also on the left side between areas 1 and 2. Massaging here affects the Wind of the stomach and spleen.

7. The seventh area is on the right side of the navel between areas 2 and 3. Massaging here affects the Wind of the liver and gall bladder.

8. The eighth and last area is on the right side between areas 3 and 4. Massaging here also affects the Wind of the intestines.

After you have finished this massage, you can massage all around the abdominal area seeking out any knots, lumps, tight or painful spots. Doing this Self-Massage regularly is one of the best gifts you could ever give yourself.

Yi Chin Ching: The Muscle-Tendon Change Classic—Part Four

I hope you were able to put all the pieces together and do last week's Muscle-Tendon Change exercises. If you found it too confusing, just work on the forms and in time the details should fall into place.

This week you'll learn some more forms. Again they are all extremely simple movements. The basic forms this week are variations of ones you learned last week.

Forms 5 – 8

You hold your arms at your sides for these four forms. On inhalation the arms are relaxed. Your armpits are rounded as if there were an egg there and your shoulders are dropped. Upon exhalation your arms are straightened and your shoulders are pushed down. The hands are squeezed in the same four patterns as in Week One.

A helpful note on squeezing the hands and feet: when squeezing the hands, spread the fingers apart and begin the squeeze at the wrists and move out to the fingertips. Squeeze the forearm next and then the upper arm. When squeezing the feet, bend the knees slightly on inhalation and straighten the legs upon exhalation as you squeeze the toes, feet, calves and thighs.

Form 5. Your palms face forward.

Form 6. Your palms face your thighs.

Form 7. Your palms face backward, behind you.

Form 8. Your palms face outward, away from your sides, as you exhale and squeeze.

In all these four forms, your arms remain at the side of your body as you squeeze.

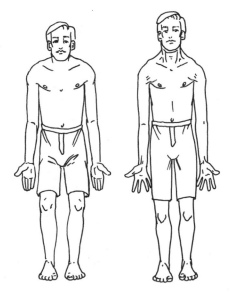

Forms 9 – 12

Form 9. The arms are held straight overhead with the palms facing out to the sides, away from each other.

Form 10. The arms are held straight overhead with the palms facing forward.

Form 11. The arms are held straight overhead. The palms face each other.

Form 12. The arms are held straight overhead. The palms face backward.

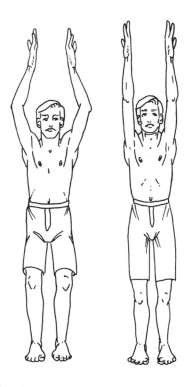

Do each form at least 3 times or do one of each in sequence at least three times. Inhale and relax your arms, elbows and shoulders. Exhale and push your arms upward and squeeze; your shoulders move in toward your ears as you do.

Forms 13 – 16

These four forms are performed with the arms held out to the sides at shoulder level. Inhale and relax arms, sinking the elbows and draw in the shoulder blades. Exhale and straighten the arms and push the shoulder blades and shoulders out to your sides.

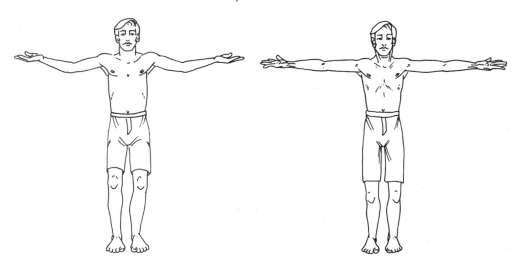

Form 13. Your arms are held at shoulder level straight out to your sides. Your palms face upward.

Form 14. Your palms face forward.

Form 15. Your palms face down.

Form 16. Your palms face backward.

Forms 1 – 16 (Variation A)

In this variation, instead of squeezing the hands, you make a fist and squeeze the fist on exhalation. Otherwise do all the forms exactly the same as taught. When inhaling allow the fist to relax and open slightly. On exhalation also open the eyes wide and glare as you learned in Week Four, Baduanjin, the Seventh Piece: Clenching the Fists and Glaring to Increase Strength. Your thumb can be either outside the fist as you would normally when you make a fist or inside your fist with the other fingers wrapped around it.

Forms 1 – 16 (Variation B)

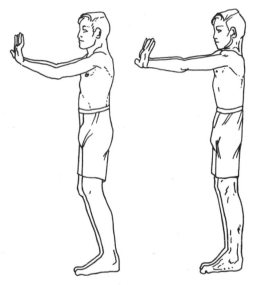

In this variation you pull back your wrist and fingers toward your shoulders as you exhale and squeeze. The wrists are held at a 90-degree angle to your forearm when relaxed, and pulled back toward your shoulder, as far as you can, when you squeeze. Otherwise the forms are identical to the previous ones. This variation can be very painful, but it is tremendously effective to lengthen and change your tendons.

The Muscle-Tendon Change Classic exercises are designed to stretch the tendons. This causes the tendons to lengthen and soften. These are wonderful exercises for tight shoulders and neck. They are good for arthritis sufferers. Keep at them, sometimes it takes a while for them to become effective. I have modified these exercises for beginning Western practitioners. There are many other forms of Yi Chin Ching. Most of them are also simple, but without a teacher present, the details of each might be too confusing.

If you apply the details and practice, you will get results—sometimes startling results. Always close a session by shaking out your hands.

A few shakes of your feet can't hurt either. Just raise one leg at the knee and shake out the foot, then shake the other foot.

Learning Yi Chin Ching from a book is probably not the best way to learn it. However, I have given you details of the practice, which are also applicable to many other forms of Chi Kung, that you would be hard pressed to find anywhere else. I wish you all success in your practice.

Sexual Kung Fu: Testicle and Ovarian Breathing–Part Three

This week we finally begin to raise the Jing Chi up the spine. This practice is essentially identical for men and women. The Jing Chi is drawn from the perineum directly into the bottom of the spine and into the sacrum. You will realize how important the numerous exercises for differentiating and strengthening the various parts of the perineum and anus are in completing this gentle exercise. You must also activate the Sacral Pump to pump the Sexual Energy up the spine.

I mentioned earlier in this book that Jing Chi—Sexual Energy—is heavier and denser than Chi. It is necessary to actually pump it up the spine, while Chi can be directed with the mind alone. It is also necessary to use the Yi Mind to hold the Jing Chi in place, like a fingertip on the end of a straw, to keep it from sinking down and out of the sacrum.

The Jing Chi actually enters the spine at a point called the sacral hiatus, which is a small opening in the sacrum about one inch above the tip of the coccyx on the outer part of the spine. If the sacral hiatus is blocked, the Jing Chi will not be able to enter the spine. It is recommended that you massage the coccyx and the lower sacrum with a silk cloth to help open the hiatus.

Testicle Breathing: Part Three

When we draw the cold Yin Jing Chi up and into the spine, we are not drawing semen up the spine. We are drawing the Essence of cold, non-aroused male sexual energy from the sperm cells. Some Western sources have misunderstood and ridiculed this technique because they believed that the semen itself was supposed to be raised up the spine and into the head. This is physically impossible and is not what is going on here. You are raising Energy generated by the sperm. The cold Yin Jing Chi is heavier and denser than the warm Yang Jing Chi that women raise in Ovarian Breathing, so this exercise might be more difficult for men than women.

1. Begin with Testicle Breathing.

2. Draw the Sexual Energy to the perineum as you learned last week.

3. Inhale and direct the Jing Chi through the "silver straw" and toward the coccyx by pulling first on the back of the perineum and the front of the anus and then on the back of the anus.

4. Pull up on the muscle between the back of the anus and the coccyx and the Jing Chi will be drawn up to and past the coccyx.

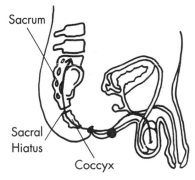

5. Use your Yi Mind to locate the opening at the bottom of the sacrum called the sacral hiatus. Direct the Jing Chi through the "silver straw" and into the sacral hiatus. It might help to gently pull in on the eye muscles to control the Sexual Energy.

6. Activate the Sacral Pump by pulling the bottom of the sacrum in toward the body and flattening and pushing the Ming Men away from the body. Activate the Cranial Pump by pulling in the chin and tightening the back of the neck and skull. This will cause the Jing Chi to rise into the sacrum.

7. Use your Yi Mind to hold the Jing Chi in the sacrum, like a finger on the "silver straw."

8. Exhale and release the Sacral and Cranial Pumps while holding the Jing Chi in the sacrum with the Yi Mind.

9. Repeat 9 times, drawing Sexual Energy from the testicles to the perineum, past the coccyx and into the sacrum. Continue to hold and accumulate the Jing Chi in the sacrum with the Yi Mind as you draw up more Sexual Energy with each breath.

10. After 9 breaths, imagine or feel that you are pouring the Jing Chi from the top of the sacrum, into the Tan Tien just below and behind the navel.

Holding the Jing Chi in place with the Yi Mind is quite simple. It doesn't require your full concentration. It is as if you can split your consciousness and use ten percent of it to hold the Jing Chi in place and the remainder of your awareness to help draw more Sexual Energy up and into the sacrum.

You might actually experience cold energy rise into your sacrum or you might experience a feeling of pins and needles. As you practice you should become more proficient with coordinating the sequential pull of the muscles in the front of the perineum, the back of the perineum, the back of the anus and up to the coccyx. Don't use force. This is a gentle exercise.

Ovarian Breathing: Part Three

The female practice is almost identical to the male practice.

1. Begin with Ovarian Breathing.

2. Draw the Sexual Energy to the perineum as you learned last week.

3. Inhale small sips of air, keep the lips of the vagina lightly closed and direct the Jing Chi through the "silver straw" and toward the coccyx by pulling on the back of the perineum and the front of the anus and then on the back of the anus.

4. Pull up on the muscle between the back of the anus and the coccyx and the Jing Chi will be drawn up to and past the coccyx.

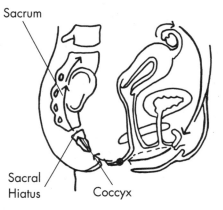

5. Use your Yi Mind to locate the opening at the bottom of the sacrum called the sacral hiatus. Direct the Jing Chi through the "silver straw" and into the sacral hiatus. It might help to gently pull in on the eye muscles to control the Sexual Energy.

6. Activate the Sacral Pump by pulling the bottom of the sacrum in toward the body and flattening and pushing the Ming Men away from the body. Activate the Cranial Pump by pulling in the chin and tightening the back of the neck and skull. This will cause the Jing Chi to rise into the sacrum.

7. Use your Yi Mind to hold the Jing Chi in the sacrum, like a finger on the "silver straw."

8. Exhale and release the Sacral and Cranial Pumps while holding the Jing Chi in the sacrum with the Yi Mind.

9. Repeat 9 times, drawing Sexual Energy from the Ovarian Palace, to the perineum, past the coccyx and into the sacrum. Continue to hold and accumulate the Jing Chi in the sacrum with the Yi Mind as you draw up more Sexual Energy with each breath.

10. After 9 breaths, imagine or feel that you are pouring the Jing Chi from the top of the sacrum, into the Tan Tien just below and behind the navel.

As mentioned, women draw up warm Yang Jing Chi which is lighter and less dense than cold Yin Jing Chi. This part of the practice might therefore be initially easier for women than men.

The Microcosmic Orbit: Part Two

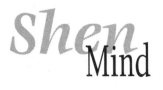

TO KEEP THINGS AS SIMPLE as possible, this week's lesson will mirror what you have been learning in the last two Sexual Kung Fu lessons. We will move the Chi to the perineum and then raise it into the sacrum. This begins the process of connecting the Functional Channel which runs down the front of the body with the Governor Channel which runs up the back.

Chi is much easier to move than Sexual Energy. So if you have been having any success with the Testicle or Ovarian Breathing, this week's Regulating the Mind exercise should be a snap. The technique is different though. The Microcosmic Orbit is concerned with circulating the Warm Current, Chi that has been heated in the stove. By this week you should be quite proficient at Warming the Stove.

Traditionally one learns to move the Chi in the Microcosmic Orbit by using the Yi Mind and breathing techniques. Remember you lead the Chi with the mind. You can't push it. However at this stage in your practice you are not yet ready to circulate Chi in the Microcosmic Orbit by mind power alone, which is actually an advanced practice. In these exercises the mind and the breath are coordinated to move the Chi.

A major addition to the technique this week is the use of both Abdominal Breathing and Reverse Breathing in the exercise. We use Abdominal Breathing to Warm the Stove and as we move Chi from the Tan Tien to the Sperm/Ovarian Palace and then to the perineum. We use Reverse Breathing to raise the Chi up the spine, this week up to the sacrum.

1. Repeat last week's lesson through Step 8: Bellows Breathing to Warm the Stove.

2. With your mind focused on the Tan Tien and your inner ears listening to your silent breathing, regulate your breath by doing a few slow Abdominal Breaths.

3. Inhale an Abdominal Breath and lower your concentration to the Sperm/Ovarian Palace as you exhale and guide the Chi to the Sperm/Ovarian Palace. Continue doing Abdominal Breathing for a minute or so as you feel this area begin to warm up.

4. Inhale an Abdominal Breath and lower your concentration to your perineum as you exhale and guide the Chi to the perineum. Maintain your concentration here for a minute or more as you continue to do Abdominal Breathing.

5. Inhale an Abdominal Breath and raise the Chi back to the Sperm/Ovarian Palace.

6. Exhale and lower the Chi back to the perineum. Do this 9 times. This is called Washing the Channel and helps to open the points on the Orbit.

7. After the final exhalation with the Chi lowered back to the perineum, pull in the lower abdomen as you inhale. Do Reverse Breathing, pulling up in sequence on the perineum, the back of the anus and the muscle connected to the coccyx, using your mind to raise the Chi up past the coccyx, into the sacral hiatus and into the sacrum.

8. Keep your concentration on the Sacrum for a minute or two as you continue to do gentle Reverse Breathing.

9. Exhale and lower the Chi back to the perineum. Inhale and raise it back to the sacrum. Wash the Channel 9 times.

10. Conclude the exercise by collecting the Energy at the navel as previously learned.

Sole Breathing

THE TAOISTS PLACED THE HIGHEST priority on "breathing from the heels." This doesn't mean that we'll now learn how to breathe with our feet. Rather it refers to the ability to draw Earth Energy or Yin Chi from the ground and up the legs.

Chi *Breath*

We will learn to draw Yin Chi into the feet, up the legs to the perineum and then return it to the Earth. We do this in coordination with Reverse Breathing.

Chi is drawn from the Earth through the point on the sole of the foot known as the Bubbling Spring (Yong Quan). It's located just behind the ball of the foot in the center of the sole. If you press on this point it is very often tender. We will learn to massage it in this week's Self-Massage Rejuvenation.

Drawing Yin Chi from the Earth will help to ground and center us. As with many of the exercises in this book, you may initially have to use your imagination to "feel" the Chi rise or descend through the legs. But many of you are probably now sufficiently advanced in the practice to actually experience the flow of Chi. Once you learn to draw Earth Energy, you will get a terrific boost in your practice. The Earth itself will give you its Energy to strengthen and support you.

1. Begin Reverse Breathing as you learned last week.

2. Inhale, contracting the lower Abdomen and pull up on the perineum and sexual organs.

3. Simultaneously feel or imagine Chi entering your feet through the Bubbling Spring point and flow to your heels and then up the back of the legs, through the calves, knees and thighs. The Chi flows from the back of both legs into the perineum.

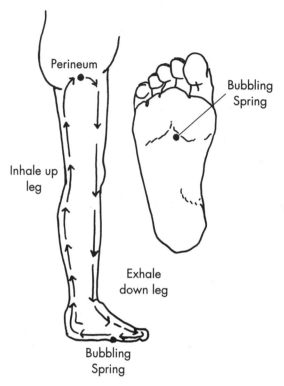

4. Exhale and expand the lower abdomen and push down on your perineum.

5. Simultaneously, lower the Chi from the perineum down the front of both legs, through your thighs, knees and ankles, over the top of your feet and toes to the Bubbling Spring on the underside of your feet, behind the ball of your foot.

6. Repeat at least 6 times per session.

This exercise becomes even more effective if you can shift your consciousness into the Earth before drawing the Yin Chi into the Bubbling Spring. The deeper you can project into the Earth, the more powerful the Yin Chi will be that rises up. This was one of the great secrets of Taoist martial artists. By tapping into the Earth they became so grounded that they could not be moved. I often saw Mantak Chia, who couldn't weigh more than 145 pounds, line up twenty people and have them all push against him. I never saw anyone even budge him. I did manage to move him once, but we were standing in a swimming pool in five feet of water at the time.

Some of you might find it easier to raise and lower the Yin Chi up and down the middle of the leg rather than up the back and down the front. You should be able to do this anyway, so try it both ways.

You can do this exercise while standing, sitting or walking.

Taoist Self-Massage Rejuvenation: Hitting to Detoxify the Legs

HITTING AND SLAPPING ARE EFFECTIVE Taoist techniques for removing toxins, increasing blood circulation, stimulating the bone marrow, softening and loosening up the muscles and tendons and clearing blockages from the Energy Channels. Hitting and slapping the legs will help to accomplish all these goals.

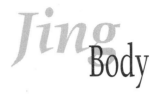

The method is again very simple: you will slap down the leg with an open palm and reverse and hit up the leg with a loosely held fist. We will hit down each leg in four separate lines: Front, inside, outside and back. You can do this standing or sitting with your legs stretched out in front of you.

1. Rub your hands together until hot. Begin with the left leg.

2. The Front Line: Slap with open left hand from the top of the left thigh, down the thigh, over the knee, down the front of the calf, past the ankle to the tips of the toes. Reverse and hit with a loosely held left fist, up from the toes to the top of the thigh.

3. The Inner Line: Slap from the top of the inner left thigh, down the inner side of the leg to the inner side of the ankle, to the big toe. Reverse and hit with the fist from the big toe back to the top of the inner thigh. Men, take care to cover or protect your genitals.

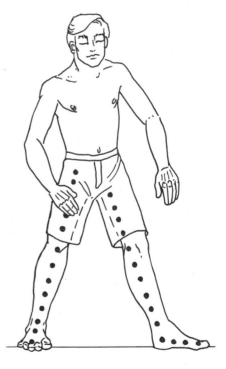

4. The Outer Line: Slap the outside of the left leg, from the hip joint down the thigh, calf and ankle to the pinkie toe. Reverse and hit up the outside of the leg with a loosely held fist.

5. The Back Line: Slap down with the left hand, from the buttocks, down the back of the thigh to the knee. Slap the back of the knees sharply at least 6 times to release toxins and sediment that accumulate there. This might initially result in raising welts or purple dots (which

are released sediment) on the back of the knee, but is quite beneficial. Continue slapping down the back of the calf to the left heel. Reverse and hit with a loosely held fist from the heel back up to the left buttock.

6. The Sole of the Foot-Bubbling Spring: Lift your left foot, pull up on your toes to stretch the muscles and tendons. Place your thumbs below the ball of the foot and locate a depression close to the center of the foot. Keeping the toes raised, massage deeply into the depression; it will probably be quite tender or tight. If it isn't, move the thumbs around until you find any tender spots and massage there. Sharply slap the bottom of the foot at least 9 times.

7. Repeat Steps 1 through 6 on the right leg and foot.

You can substitute a sock filled with dry beans (mung and black beans are recommended) in place of the open hand and fist.

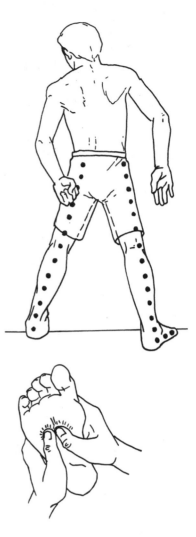

Tao In: Part One

Tao In exercises are the Taoist equivalent of Hatha Yoga. They seem to have originated as sets of calisthenics combining physical movement and breathing more than two thousand years ago. There is a vast body of exercises that are called Tao In; some are quite simple and others are quite intricate. We'll stay away from the latter. There are some sources in English that have described and illustrated many Tao In forms. However, like Yi Chin Ching, it is the details that often are not obvious that really make the exercises work. By and large these details have never been revealed in English.

This week and next week we will concentrate on Tao In exercises for the legs and the psoas muscles. The psoas muscles of the lower back are among the most important muscle groups in the body. Many of the exercises in this book, including the Sexual Kung Fu and Microcosmic Orbit, benefit greatly from strengthened psoas muscles. They are crucial for the proper working of the Sacral Pump.

The psoas muscles (psoas Major and Minor) connect to all the vertebrae in the lower thoracic and lumbar areas of the spine. Another segment (Iliopsoas) runs down to the pelvis and thigh bones. When the psoas group of muscles is relaxed, its broad flat surface offers support for all the organs of the lower abdomen. The psoas draws the legs forward during walking and largely determines body posture by setting the tilt of the pelvis in relation to the rest of the body. Its normal function is involved with the entire working of the back, hips and pelvic area.

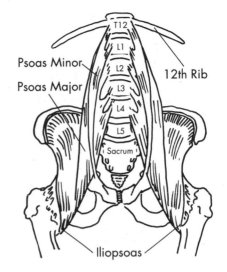

If the psoas muscles become shortened, they can pull the whole body out of balance. If just one side of the psoas muscles gets shortened, it results in muscles on both sides of the body working to compensate for the one-sided pull. This can result in many negative side effects such as tilting of the pelvis to one side, rigidity in the thigh bones, stiffness and tenderness in the lower back and a whole host of ankle and foot problems.

Tension, fear and cold energy cause the psoas muscles to contract. They are next to the kidneys, the seat of cold Water Energy. Too much cold energy in the kidneys causes the psoas muscles to tighten and shorten. When doing the Tao In exercises, it is important therefore to warm up the kidneys. This is accomplished by doing the Heart Healing Sound H-A-W-W-W-W-W-W, which will cause heat to escape the heart through the pericardium. Mentally draw this heat back toward the spine and it will sink down toward the kidneys and warm them up. This in turn will warm up the psoas muscles which causes them to relax.

The psoas muscles are also intimately related to the proper functioning of the diaphragm. If the psoas are warm and supple, it is easier to breathe deeply. They are also closely connected to the latissimus dorsi muscles that spread out from the upper spine to the shoulders. The psoas muscles are an important bridge between the lower and upper body.

Most of these exercises are performed while sitting or lying on the floor or ground. A firm surface is required. They cannot be properly done on a bed or soft, yielding surface. So finding a place to practice is the first step. They don't require a lot of space, just enough to lie down and spread your arms or legs out a little bit.

Tao In #1: Warming the Psoas

This one can actually be done standing, sitting or lying down. I'll describe the prone position but the method is the same for all positions.

1. Lie down flat on your back with your legs straight out and your arms at your side. Relax and do some slow Abdominal Breaths.

2. Do the Heart Healing Sound H-A-W-W-W-W-W-W as you exhale. As you do it feel your heart relax and seem to sink deeper into your chest (tension causes the heart to rise closer to the surface of the chest). Do at least 6 Heart Healing Sounds.

3. Feel heat coming out of the heart. Mentally draw the heat to your spine.

4. Feel the heat descend the spine to the two kidneys. Feel the kidneys begin to warm up.

5. The heat spreads out from the kidneys down into the lower back. This is the region of the psoas muscles.

6. Feel your lower back warm up and relax.

7. If necessary, do more Heart Healing Sounds.

Tao In #2: Opening the Groin

Very often the muscles around the groin and upper thigh (especially the iliopsoas) and the tendons grow tight and stiff, restricting normal movement. Tightness in this region limits mobility when walking and during sexual intercourse. Here is a simple Tao In exercise to open and relax this area, which the Taoists call the *kua*.

1. Sit up on the floor.

2. Your legs are open with your knees bent out to your sides, and the soles of both feet touching each other in front of you. You form sort of a diamond shape with your legs. Taoists call this the butterfly position.

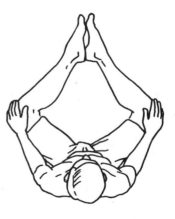

3. Place a hand palm down on each knee. Unless you are very relaxed and supple, chances are each knee is raised an inch or two off the ground.

4. Use your hands to lightly push down and bounce your knees down to the ground.

5. Repeat at least 9 times. The knees should bounce back up of their own accord each time. Don't use too much force, especially if there is a lot of pain on the sides of the groin. In time the pain and stiffness will pass. The closer you pull your feet in toward the groin, the more tension you will experience as you exercise.

Tao In #3: The Psoas Stretch

This is a multi-step exercise designed to stretch the psoas muscles so that one side of the psoas shouldn't be longer than the other side. This exercise is performed while lying on the floor. The legs are again held in the Butterfly position, a diamond shape with the soles of the feet touching. However, this time your legs are raised off the ground. This is where it is important to pay attention to details. It is important that when you raise your legs, you also raise your buttocks off the ground (activate the Sacral Pump) and flatten your lower back (sacrum) and middle back into the ground. The exercise is otherwise simple.

Variation A:

1. Lie flat on the ground. Raise your legs, spread out your knees and bring the soles of your feet together in the diamond shaped Butterfly position. Your knees will be about a foot and a half off the ground at a 45-degree angle to the ground.

2. Raise your buttocks off the floor and flatten your lower and middle back into the ground.

3. Keeping the back of your head on the ground, move your arms down between your legs and grab the top of the calves, just below the knees, with each hand.

4. Do Abdominal Breathing as you hold on to the top of the calves to prevent them from falling as you keep your buttocks raised off the ground. You should feel a real pull in the lower back as gravity tries to do its job.

5. Hold for up to 30 seconds.

Variation B:

This exercise is identical to *Variation A* except the hands are moved down to hold the ankles.

Variation C:

Again identical to *Variation A* except the hands are moved down to hold the soles of the feet.

Variation D:

This exercise starts from the same position as *Variation C*. The legs are in the Butterfly position, with the buttocks raised off the ground and the lower and middle back pushed into the ground.

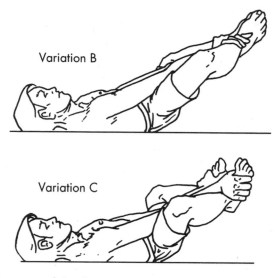

Variation B

Variation C

Each hand is holding the bottom of the foot.

1. Inhale an Abdominal Breath.

2. Exhale and push the bottom of your feet against the palms of the hand, as if you were trying to straighten your legs. You will feel a powerful stretch in the psoas region.

3. Inhale and relax.

4. Repeat at least 3 times per session.

Tao In #4: The Tao In Sit Up

We will learn two forms of the Tao In Sit Up, Variation A with one knee raised and Variation B with both knees raised.

In order to stretch the psoas muscles, the buttocks are again raised and the lower and middle back flattened into the ground as we perform these exercises. This is crucial to making them work.

Variation A: Tao In Sit Up with One Knee Raised

1. Lie flat on your back and inhale an Abdominal Breath. Raise and bend your right knee and bring the heel of your right foot up to your buttocks with the sole of your foot right on the ground. Your left leg is stretched out straight.

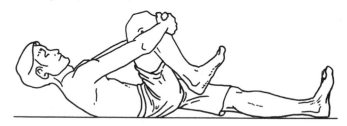

2. Interlock your fingers and clasp both hands around the top of your right knee.

3. Raise your buttocks off the ground and flatten your sacrum and middle back into the ground.

4. Begin the sit up by exhaling and pulling your right knee toward your head. Your left leg remains stretched straight out with the foot held upright.

5. Raise your head and shoulders off the ground but keep your shoulders and your neck straight. Do not bend your neck as you raise up.

6. It is not necessary to raise your head and shoulders more than a few inches. Your right knee does not touch your chin as you pull on it.

7. Exhale and relax. Repeat at least 3 times per session.

8. Repeat as above with left knee bent and right leg straight.

Variation B: Tao In Sit Up with Both Knees Raised

1. Lie flat on your back with both knees raised and bent and the heels of both feet tucked into your butt with the soles flat on the floor. Inhale an Abdominal Breath.

2. Interlock the fingers of both hands and clasp around the top of both knees.

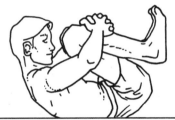

3. Exhale and raise your buttocks off the ground and flatten your middle back into the ground.

4. Pull both knees toward your head.

5. Simultaneously raise your head and shoulders and try to bring your chin as close to your knees as you can. You can bend your neck this time.

6. Inhale and relax.

7. Do at least 3 per session.

Sexual Kung Fu: Testicle and Ovarian Breathing–Part Four

As the Jing Chi rises up the spine, it is converted into Chi. The analogy, again, is like fuel being converted into usable energy. The conversion process begins in the sacrum. It continues as the Sexual Energy rises up the spine past the Ming Men and is completed by the time it reaches the point on the spine opposite the solar plexus, known as the Chi Chung or T-11 point. This week you will learn how to raise the Jing Chi from the sacrum to the Chi Chung.

As the Sexual Energy rises and is converted into Chi, it becomes lighter and less dense and thus easier to move. It's getting the Jing Chi to begin to rise that's the most difficult part. Once you get it to begin flowing backward, it gets easier rather than harder to move.

This week's practice is identical for men and women, so there will not be a separate section for each.

1. Repeat last week's practice through Step 8, holding the Jing Chi at the sacrum.

2. Draw more Jing Chi, from either the testicles or the ovaries, to the perineum.

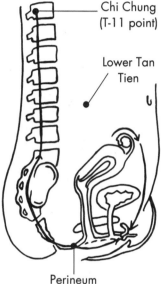

Chi Chung
(T-11 point)

Lower Tan
Tien

Perineum

3. Inhale and direct the Jing Chi through the "silver straw" toward the coccyx by pulling up on the per-ineum, the front of the anus, the back of the anus and the muscle between the back of the anus and the coccyx and the Jing Chi will be drawn up to and past the coccyx.

4. Direct the Jing Chi through the "silver straw" into the sacral hiatus. Pull in gently on the eye muscles to aid in drawing up the Jing Chi.

5. Activate the Sacral pump by pulling in the bottom of the sacrum and flattening and pushing the lower and middle back outward away from the body. Activate the Cranial Pump by pulling in the chin and tight-ening the back of the neck and skull. This will cause the Jing Chi to rise up the sacrum.

6. Continue to draw the Jing Chi up the back in the "silver straw" to the Chi Chung (T-11 point) opposite the solar plexus.

7. Use your Yi Mind to hold the Jing Chi at the Chi Chung and draw more Sexual Energy from the testicles or ovaries.

8. Repeat a total of 9 times, then pour the Jing Chi from the Chi Chung into your Tan Tien to finish the exercise.

The Microcosmic Orbit: Part Three

THIS WEEK WE WILL RAISE the Chi up the spine to the Ming Men behind the navel, and then to the Chi Chung behind the solar plexus.

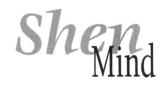

The Chi Chung is also known as the adrenal gland energy point. The adrenal glands sit on top of the two kidneys and the Chi Chung (T-11) lies right between them. The adrenal glands are complex endocrine glands that secrete a number of hormones. The outer part of the adrenal glands known as the adrenal cortex is essential to life. Through hormonal secretion it regulates the metabolism of salt, water, carbohydrates, protein and fat in the body. It also helps to regulate the body's reaction to stress and in proper sexual functioning by secreting sexual steroids. The inner part of the adrenal glands, known as the adrenal medulla, produce two hormones, adrenaline and noradrenaline (epinephrine and norepinephrine), which are famous for controlling the "fight or flight" reaction by stimulating or reducing the heart rate, blood pressure and breathing.

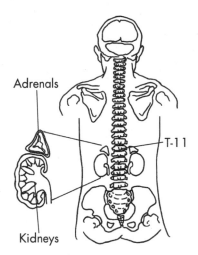

The Taoists believe that when the Chi Chung is blocked, you feel that life is a burden. When it is open, you experience the sensation of freedom. If you are feeling tired or weak, the Chi Chung adrenal point is an excellent place to focus on to renew your energy.

1. Practice what you have previously learned in the Regulating the Mind exercises up to and including Warming the Stove.

2. Place your attention on the Tan Tien and listen with your "inner ears" as you silently do a few Abdominal Breaths.

3. Inhale an Abdominal Breath. Exhale and lower your concentration to the Sperm/Ovarian Palace. Do a few Abdominal Breaths and feel your Sperm/Ovarian Palace begin to warm up.

4. Inhale an Abdominal Breath. Exhale and lower your concentration to your perineum. Do a few more Abdominal Breaths.

5. Do a final Abdominal Breath. On the exhalation, contract the lower abdomen and hold it.

6. Inhale a Reverse Breath contracting the lower Abdomen even more. Pull up in sequence on the perineum, the back of the anus and the muscle connected to the coccyx.

7. Simultaneously use your mind to guide the Chi up through the sacral hiatus, through your sacrum and up to the Ming Men point opposite your navel. Keep your concentration on the Ming Men for about a minute as you continue doing gentle Reverse Breathing.

8. Exhale and lower the Chi back to the perineum. Inhale a Reverse Breath, pull up on the back of the anus and coccyx and raise the Chi back to the Ming Men. Wash the Channel in this fashion 9 times.

9. On the final exhalation, lower the Chi back to the perineum, then inhale, pull up and raise the Chi to the Ming Men. Without exhaling, take another Reverse inhalation of air and raise the Chi up to the Chi Chung (T-11).

10. Maintain your concentration on the Chi Chung for a minute or two as you do a gentle Reverse Breath.

11. Exhale and lower the Chi down to the Ming Men. Inhale a Reverse Breath and raise it back to the Chi Chung. Wash the Channel 9 times.

12. Finish the exercise by collecting the Energy at the navel.

Chi Chung Breathing

ACTIVATING THE CHI CHUNG (T-11) acts as a mini-pump to send Chi farther up the spine. As we begin the final four weeks of the 100 Days of Practice, it is necessary that we develop this ability.

Chi Breath

Chi Chung Breathing will help to open blockages in the spine and increase your ability to raise Chi all the way up your spine. It also helps to open the Solar Plexus Point on the Functional Channel. This exercise is a variation of Reverse Breathing.

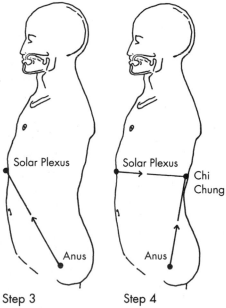

1. Do a few Abdominal Breaths. On the final exhalation, contract the lower abdomen.

2. Inhale a Reverse Breath, pulling in the lower abdomen even more.

3. Simultaneously, push up your anus toward your solar plexus (the pit of your stomach) on the Functional Channel.

4. Hold for a second then pull in the solar plexus toward your back and push up your anus toward the Chi Chung Point on your spine.

Step 3

Step 4

5. Hold the pull for a second or two, or longer if you can.

6. Relax the anus, exhale and expand the lower abdomen.

7. Repeat at least 3 times per session. Do more if you can.

As you do Chi Chung Breathing, you might feel Energy shoot up your spine and flow into your neck and head. If this happens, use your mind to lower the Chi down your spine to the Ming Men and from there pour it into your Tan Tien area (Sea of Chi) as you exhale.

Taoist Self-Massage Rejuvenation: Massaging the Solar Plexus

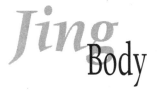

As you were doing the previous exercise, Chi Chung Breathing, you might have noticed some tightening or tension in the solar plexus region.

The solar plexus is located about an inch and one-half to two inches below the bottom of the sternum (breastbone). You should already be familiar with this point because it is where you place your fingertips when you do the Spleen Healing Sound which you learned in Week Five. The Spleen Healing Sound, W-H-O-O-O-O-O-O, is extremely helpful in relieving tension in the solar plexus area. However, this is a point that can accumulate a great deal of toxins, tightness and stress and requires massaging to fully release and relax it.

The Solar Plexus Point is called the Chung Kung in Chinese. It is often referred to in the West as the "pit of the stomach." It is located on the Functional Channel which runs down the front of the body, between the Heart and Navel Points. Massaging this point will have a beneficial effect on the spleen, pancreas, stomach and liver. The Solar Plexus Point also controls the body's aura, the electromagnetic field around the body. In addition, the Solar Plexus Point determines the location of the Middle Tan Tien, which is used by Taoists in advanced Internal Alchemy practices, which are well beyond the scope of this book.

1. Bring the back of both hands together in front of your body.

2. Press into the solar plexus area (pit of the stomach) with the index, middle and ring fingers of both hands.

3. Massage with a circular motion at least 9 times clockwise and 9 times counter-clockwise.

At first use light pressure. As you progress, you can increase the pressure. With practice, you will feel the Solar Plexus Point relax as you massage it.

This is a good massage to do in conjunction with Massaging the Lower Rib Cage and Diaphragm that you learned in Week Two. You haven't forgotten it yet, have you? You shouldn't. It's very good for you.

Seeing the Human Aura

Most people cannot see auras without special training. Gaining the ability to see the human aura is very popular among Chi Kung practitioners in China. The practice can become quite complex. I studied with one Chi Kung Master who could see all sorts of colors in the aura and diagnose patients based on the condition of their aura. Here is a simple exercise he taught me to see the human aura. It is easiest to do with the help of a partner, but it can be done with total strangers if the conditions are right.

1. Station your partner in front of a white wall, screen or surface. If white is not available, the lighter the background is, the easier it is to see the aura.

2. Stand about ten feet away and look at a point about an inch above your partner's head.

3. Don't stare too hard, just let your eyes relax.

4. In a short period of time you should see something around the edges of your partner's head. It might look like a fuzzy shadow or like heat shimmering off a hot highway surface. It might only be an inch or two high or it might surround the whole head extending out a foot or more. It might be colorless or it could be any color of the rainbow.

The idea is to see something. If you do, most people realize that they have experienced this phenomenon many times before but had simply paid it no mind. Once you get the hang of it, the aura is pretty easy to see. Be aware that auras seem to shift and appear and disappear. This is especially true if you try to stare right at them. Try to look above or to the side of it.

Everybody has an electromagnetic field. It can be photographed using Kirlian photography. Again this is science, not mysticism.

You can do this exercise alone using a large mirror with a white or light-colored surface behind you. To see the aura of someone who is not aware of what you are doing, your best opportunity will come when watching a speaker address a group of people. If the speaker is standing in front of a light-colored background, you should have no problem seeing the aura. I remember the first time I did. I was watching a lawyer sum up before a jury in a criminal case. As I watched him I could clearly see a reddish golden aura around his head. He made a strong legal point and then turned to his left while the aura continued moving to his right. I told my teacher about this. He smiled and said, "Now you got it."

Some people cannot see auras no matter how much they practice. If you are one of these people, do not despair. You have lots of other exercises in this book to keep you busy.

Protecting the Aura

The aura is just a name for the electromagnetic field that surrounds all living things. Whether we can see it or not, our own electromagnetic field interacts with and overlaps the electromagnetic field of others whenever we are in people's company. These aura fields are affected by our own thoughts and feelings as well as those of others. Brain waves have minute electrical charges that can alter the electromagnetic field of the aura.

Taoist martial artists use the aura in a number of ways to defeat their opponents. The major technique involves extending one's own aura to envelop the opponent. Once your adversary is inside your energy field, you can sense his or her movements before they happen.

The Solar Plexus Point controls the aura. It is good to have it opened and not blocked. When it is closed or tight, you can experience worry and panic. When it is open, you feel daring and can take risks. However, if the Solar Plexus Point is too open, and you are sensitive by nature, it may become impossible to shield out the mental and emotional thoughts and feelings of others when you are in their company and you can feel overwhelmed, lost or inadequate.

You should be able to make your own choice of how much you want to be open to another person or group of people. Here's how to do it.

1. Imagine a shield in front of your solar plexus. It can take any shape you want it to, and if you are visually inclined, have any design or inscription you like. (Your initials will do just fine.)

2. When your shield is in front of your solar plexus, you literally shield this point and your aura condenses. This protects you from being affected by the thoughts and feelings of other people.

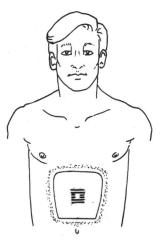

3. Raise or lower your shield as much as you wish, to determine the degree of interaction and intimacy you desire.

Tao In: Part Two

We continue this week with Tao In exercises for the legs and psoas muscles. The set you will learn this week is among my personal favorites. All of them are performed lying on your back. The key to them all is to keep your buttocks raised off the floor, push the lower and middle back into the ground and practice Abdominal Breathing. The active part of the exercises coincides with the exhalation of breath.

Tao In #5: Push Out the Elbows and Squeeze the Knees

1. Lie on your back with your legs raised off the ground and feet together in the Butterfly position.

2. Place both arms between your legs, raised above the mid-line of your body, with the palms of both hands together.

3. Push out both elbows until each is touching a knee, bring the knees slightly together, if necessary, to bring into contact with your elbows.

4. Inhale an Abdominal Breath and remain relaxed.

5. Exhale slowly and simultaneously try to squeeze the knees together as you push out with the elbows to prevent the knees from moving more than an inch or two. Raise your buttocks off the ground.

6. Inhale and relax, lowering your buttocks to the ground.

7. Repeat at least 3 times per session.

Tao In #6: Push Up the Knees

1. Lie on your back with your legs together but off the ground with your knees bent at a 90-degree angle so that your legs are L shaped off the ground (calves are horizontal to the ground).

2. Clasp your hands around the top of both knees with fingers interlocked.

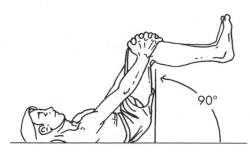

90°

3. Inhale an Abdominal Breath and remain relaxed.

4. Exhale slowly and raise your buttocks off the ground as you push your knees straight up toward the sky while you simultaneously restrain them by pulling downward with your hands.

5. Inhale, relax and lower your buttocks.

6. Repeat at least 3 times per session.

Tao In #7: Push the Knees Toward the Head

1. Lie on your back with your knees raised as in Tao In #6. However, in addition, cross the ankles.

2. Raise the tip of your tongue to the roof of your mouth behind the teeth.

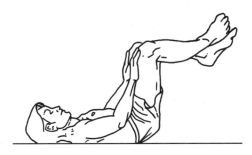

3. Place the palm of each hand, with fingers pointing upward, about two-thirds the way up each thigh so that your fingertips just touch your knees.

4. Inhale an Abdominal Breath and remain relaxed.

5. Exhale, raise your buttocks off the ground and try to push your knees toward your head while you simultaneously prevent this by pushing your hands against your thighs.

6. Inhale, relax and lower your buttocks.

7. Repeat at least 3 times per session.

Tao In #8: Pull the Knees Apart

1. Lie on your back with your legs together but off the ground with your knees bent at a 90-degree angle so that your legs are L shaped off the ground (calves are horizontal to the ground). This is the same starting position as in Tao In #6.

2. Clasp your hands around the top of both knees with fingers interlocked.

3. Inhale an Abdominal Breath and remain relaxed.

4. Exhale slowly and raise your buttocks off the ground.

5. Simultaneously try to pull your knees apart (outward) while you prevent them from moving more than a few inches with your arms and clasped hands.

6. Inhale, relax and lower your buttocks.

7. Repeat at least 3 times per session.

Sexual Kung Fu: Testicle and Ovarian Breathing–Part Five

This week you draw the Jing Chi up the "silver straw" all the way to the top of the head as you learn to complete the practice of Testicle and Ovarian Breathing.

There is actually quite a bit of work to do this week. It could be that some of you will want to spread this week's lesson out over two weeks. As I've been saying all along, there is no need to rush. You just have to practice every day.

In the previous four weeks of Testicle/Ovarian Breathing, you learned to activate or move to only one body point at a time. In the first lesson we activated the testicles or the ovaries. In the second lesson you brought the Sexual Energy down to the perineum. In the third lesson you learned to draw the Jing Chi through the sacral hiatus and up the sacrum. Last week you learned to draw the Sexual Energy up the spine to the Chi Chung point opposite the solar plexus.

This week we will raise the Sexual Energy to two different points: the Jade Pillow at the base of the skull and finally to the Crown Point (Pai Hui) at the top of the skull. Until you reach the crown, the exercise is basically identical for men and women.

Men raise cool Yin Jing Chi to the brain. It is safe to leave this cold energy in the head. It will not harm the brain. Women, however, raise warm Yang Jing Chi to the head and this warm Energy must be lowered out of the brain at the end of the exercise, down to the Tan Tien.

Raising unaroused Sexual Energy to the head has a soothing, rejuvenating effect on the brain. These practices lay the groundwork for raising aroused Sexual Energy to the brain, which you will learn in Week Thirteen.

The practice of Testicle and Ovarian Breathing was often used by celibate monks and nuns especially among the Buddhists, who adopted these practices from the Taoists. The Taoists believed that unless you knew how to channel your Sexual Energy, celibacy was an unhealthy lifestyle that often resulted in deviant behavior, neuroses and delusions of moral and spiritual superiority.

Human sexuality is part of the natural scheme of things. To the Taoists, denying this part separates you from nature's way. If one seeks celibacy for a spiritual purpose, this is a worthy endeavor, but this will not stop your sexual organs from working, they will just have no outlet. This is where trouble often arises. The Taoists found that the practices you've been learning for five weeks now were the absolute best way to cope with the stress of celibacy and, at the same time, benefit by drawing the converted Sexual Energy to the brain.

Ovarian Breathing was a widespread practice among Taoist and Buddhist nuns. It was found that by diligent practice, along with doing many of the other exercises in this book, especially the Stilling the Mind practices, the menses cycle actually stopped. They called this "slaying the Red Dragon." This meant that the nuns did not lose Jing monthly as other women do.

For my female readers, be aware of the fantastic potential of this teaching. By this I don't mean I want you to start practicing like nuns. A Taoist nun would practice Ovarian Kung Fu big time to get her monthly bleeding to stop. Her body would rejuvenate to that of a young girl and her breasts would shrink. Now that's a lot for anyone to ask of you.

The potential I'm talking about is the ability to conserve your Energy. Even if it's only a little bit each month. Ovarian Breathing will help you to conserve some Original Jing each month that would otherwise run out of your body with your blood. The longer you save your Original Jing, the longer you will live.

Remember we were born with a fixed amount of Original Jing. Taoists believe Original Jing is stored in the kidneys. The kidneys "wash" our blood. Each month a little leaks out with the menses or, for a man, when you ejaculate. Jing is our Essence, composed of all the body's fluids and hormones. Sexual Jing is an adult's most powerful form of Essence and is referred to throughout this book as Jing Chi—Sexual Energy.

As Jing Chi rises up the spine it is converted into a special form of Chi that has a rejuvenating effect on the spinal column, nervous system and brain. This special Chi is also referred to as Jing Chi, but it has been converted from Essence that the body can store into Energy the body can use. It is much thicker and denser than the Chi that you circulate in the Microcosmic Orbit exercises. That Chi is Heated in the Stove prior to circulation. It moves easily when led by the mind and pumped by the breath.

In Testicle/Ovarian Breathing, the Jing Chi is unaroused. It must be sucked up to the brain through the imaginary "Silver Straw" I've had you visualize, with little sips of air and contractions of the testicles or the lips of the vagina.

It can be held in place by using an imaginary finger. If you could see the Jing Chi with your Inner Eyes, it might appear as a dense white fog rising up your spine like whipped cream coming out of a can's nozzle.

When your brain is filled with Jing Chi, in time it leads to the secretion of a honey-like substance that drips down from the pituitary area and seems to pass right through the roof of the mouth to the tip of the raised tongue. This substance had a lot of different names. Heavenly Nectar or just plain Nectar were probably the most popular. Don't expect this to happen this week. It could take years or it could happen tomorrow. Don't expect anything. That is the true Taoist attitude. If you expect something then you have already begun to formulate what it is you expect to happen. Having some preconceived notion about what should happen separates you from what is actually happening and might lead you to miss it when it really does happen, because that was not what you expected. Act as if it doesn't matter whether it happens or not. This is the meaning of "being without desire."

Testicle and Ovarian Breathing are profoundly helpful exercises in learning to gain control of our own Sexual Energy as well as our sex drive. As the Taoists say, "You either control your sex or you are controlled by sex." Men will find that Testicle Breathing tends to cool off an over-active sexual imagination. This helps you reign in the powerful Yang sex drive with peaceful, gentle and soothing Yin Sexual Energy. In time you gain the ability to detach from the powerful spell that sex weaves upon us. This doesn't mean that you will be less sexy (you will probably be more sexy), or that you will enjoy sex less (you will probably enjoy it more). It does mean you will waste less time and energy thinking about or fantasizing about sex. This will give you more time to practice Taoist Yoga.

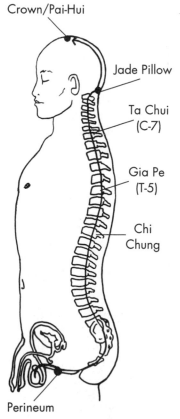

Crown/Pai-Hui

Jade Pillow

Ta Chui
(C-7)

Gia Pe
(T-5)

Chi
Chung

Perineum

Men:

1. Repeat last week's exercise through Step 8. You are using the Yi Mind like a finger, to hold the Sexual Energy in place at the Chi Chung Point.

2. Return your attention to your testicles. Inhale and gently pull up your testicles and simultaneously lightly contract the perineum, the front of the anus, the back of

the anus and the muscle between the back of the anus and the coccyx and guide the Sexual Energy through the "Silver Straw" past the perineum. Guide the Jing Chi through the sacral hiatus and activate the sacral and cranial pumps as the Sexual Energy rises past the sacrum and Chi Chung, up the back and up the neck to the Jade Pillow (Yu Chen) at the base of the skull. This is also the general location of the cranial pump. Repeat a total of 9 times.

3. Holding the Sexual Energy at the Jade Pillow, return your concentration to your testicles and repeat the process drawing the cool Yin Jing Chi all the way up to the top of the brain, the Crown Point or Pai Hui. The proper location of this point is located by imagining a line going over the top of the head connecting the highest point of each ear. This line is intersected by another line drawn straight back over the top of the head from the tip of the nose. The Crown Point is sort of in the middle of the skull.

4. Repeat a total of 9 times.

5. Spiral the Jing Chi in the head. Use your Yi Mind to make 36 horizontal circles inside the brain, clockwise (from the front to the right side and back then around to the left side

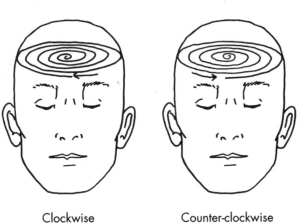

Clockwise   Counter-clockwise

and back to the front again). Reverse and do 24 counter-clockwise revolutions. This Energy can be left in the head.

Women:

1. Repeat last week's exercise through Step 8. You are using the Yi Mind like a finger, to hold the Sexual Energy in place at the Chi Chung Point.

2. Return your attention to your ovaries and Ovarian Palace. Inhale short sips of air and gently close the lips of your vagina while simultaneously lightly contracting your perineum, the front of the anus, the back of the anus and the muscle between the back of the anus and the coccyx and guide the Sexual Energy through the "Silver Straw" past the perineum. Guide the Jing Chi through the sacral hiatus and activate the sacral and cranial pumps as the Sexual Energy rises past the sacrum and Chi Chung to the Jade Pillow (Yu Chen) at the base of the skull.

This is also the general location of the cranial pump. Repeat a total of 9 times.

3. Holding the Sexual Energy at the Jade Pillow, return your concentration to your ovaries and Ovarian Palace and repeat the process drawing the warm Yang Jing Chi all the way up to the top of the brain, the Crown Point or Pai Hui. The proper location of this point is located by imagining a line going over the top of the head connecting the highest point of each ear. This line is intersected by another line drawn straight back over the top of the head from the tip of the nose. The Crown Point is in the middle of the skull.

4. Repeat a total of 9 times.

5. Spiral the Jing Chi in the head. Use your Yi Mind to make 36 horizontal circles inside the brain, counter-clockwise (from the front to the left side and back then around to the right side and back to the front again). Reverse and do 24 clockwise revolutions.

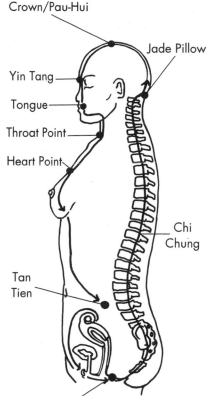

6. Raise the tip of your tongue to the roof of your mouth. Find the most comfortable spot for your tongue. Allow the Sexual Energy to flow down from your brain, from the Third Eye Point down through your raised tongue down the throat to the Heart Point at the center of your sternum (breastbone).

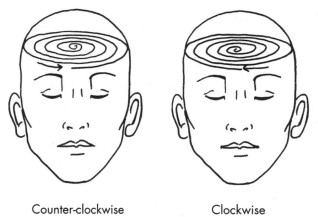

Counter-clockwise   Clockwise

7. Pause at the Heart Point and feel the Sexual Energy expand and transform into smiling, loving energy. This feeling expands through your chest and into your breasts.

8. Swallow and direct the loving Jing Chi down and into your Tan Tien below and slightly behind your navel.

Both Men and Women:

As I mentioned at the beginning of this section you may want to take two weeks to do this week's lesson. For one week (or for a few days) raise the Sexual Energy up to the Jade Pillow. The next week raise it up to the Pai Hui Crown Point. There really is no hurry, you have the rest of your life to finish this work.

Once you become proficient in doing this exercise, you should be able to draw the Jing Chi up the Silver Straw all the way from the testicles/ovaries to the top of your head in one breath. But this will never happen if you don't practice.

The Microcosmic Orbit: Part Four

Shen Mind

WE WILL BRING THE CHI all the way up the Governor Channel to the Crown Point. To a large extent this mirrors the work in this week's Sexual Kung Fu section. Chi is easier to move than Jing Chi, so this week's lesson should be easy for all.

We will be moving the Chi to the Jade Pillow at the base of the skull. As the Chi rises from the Chi Chung (T-11) to the Jade Pillow, it passes through two other points on the spine that you should be aware of. The first is the Gia Pe (T-5), located directly opposite the Heart Center, between the shoulder blades. Although the Chi must pass through this point, we don't concentrate on it because doing so has a tendency to heat up the heart and surrounding pericardium, resulting in irritability, impatience or worse. Don't worry about it, as you progress in the Microcosmic Orbit you can come back to this point and gauge your own reaction. Concentrating on this spot helps activate the heart and thymus gland. When this point is closed, you feel bogged down, hopeless, depressed and chaotic. When it is open, you have a feeling of freedom and an awareness of the importance of the higher virtues (kindness, respect, honesty, bravery, fairness, compassion) in your life.

The next point you pass through is the Ta Chui (C-7), just below the large vertebrae at the base of the neck. I debated whether to have you concentrate on this point, not only for the Microcosmic Orbit, but in this week's Sexual Kung Fu lesson. Some sources use it to open the Governor Channel. Others do not. It is not a dangerous spot, so concentrating on it will not harm you. One consideration was to keep things as simple as possible. Another is that it is better to open the Microcosmic Orbit first before spending a lot of time on the C-7 because Chi tends to get diverted at this point into the shoulders and arms. The Ta Chui is a major nerve center for Energy traveling to the arms and legs. Blockages here redirect the flow of Chi away from the head and into the extremities. If you are sending Chi (or Jing Chi) up your spine and when it reaches the bottom of your neck, it just seems to disappear and not travel up into your head, this is what is happening. If you experience this problem, spend time concentrating on your C-7. Otherwise be aware that Chi is passing through it on the way to the Jade Pillow. When this point is closed down you experience stubbornness, denial or feelings of inadequacy and not fitting in. When it is open, you feel a greater sense of connection with humanity.

The first point we will definitely work with this week is the Jade Pillow at the base of the skull. This area encompasses the cerebellum and the medulla. Both are parts of the brain and control major functions such as breathing, heartbeat and muscle coordination. It is also the back part of the cranial pump.

When the Jade Pillow is closed or blocked, energy gets stuck in the upper brain resulting in increased pressure in the brain and neck pains. This results in distraction, an inability to concentrate or meditate, and feeling suffocated. When this point is open, you experience and project inspiration.

The next point is the Crown Point, the Pai Hui (also known as the Ni Wan). This point connects with the pineal gland three inches below the crown. The pineal gland is most important in Taoist Yoga. It is the dwelling place of our Spirit (our immortal self), it controls our ability to see within ourselves (our inner eyesight), and allows us to see auras. Together with the pituitary gland (the Yin Tang, which we will reach next week) and the thalamus and hypothalamus glands, it makes up the Crystal Palace, the location of spiritual illumination.

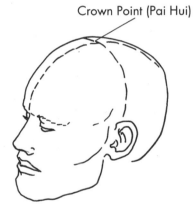

Crown Point (Pai Hui)

When the Crown Point is closed down, you could experience headaches, erratic mood swings, delusions or illusions and feeling that you are a victim or slave to others. When this point is open, you experience happiness or joyousness that radiates out to others, you may receive guidance from higher forces (in your brain or in the universe), see auras or have out-of-body experiences.

An important point of information, when guiding Energy from the base of the skull (Jade Pillow) to the top of the head (Pai Hui): be sure that you do not move the Chi to the back of the head rather than the top of the head. If you only raise the Chi to the back of the head, it can get stuck there, resulting in an end to your progress and possibly years of delay. Many people may already suffer from this problem of Energy stuck in the back of the head. The solution is to move it all the way to the Crown, and once you complete it, to circulate the Chi in the Microcosmic Orbit.

1. Repeat the meditation as you've learned it through last week. We begin with the Chi at the Chi Chung (T-11) Point.

2. Inhale a Reverse Breath, pull up on the back of the anus and coccyx and use your Yi Mind to direct the Energy upward through the spine, past the Gia Pe (T-5) and Ta Chui (C-7), up the neck to the base of the skull (Jade Pillow).

3. Keep your concentration on the Jade Pillow for at least a minute as you do gentle Reverse Breathing.

4. Exhale and lower the Chi and your point of concentration to the Chi Chong (T-11). Inhale a Reverse Breath and raise it again to the Jade Pillow. Wash the Channel 9 times.

5. Inhale a Reverse Breath, pull up on the back of the anus and coccyx and use your Yi Mind to direct the Energy up the back of your head, then forward to the Crown point.

6. Keep your concentration on the Crown Point for at least a minute as you do gentle Reverse Breathing.

7. Exhale and lower the Chi and your point of concentration to the Jade Pillow. Inhale a Reverse Breath and raise it again to the Crown Point. Wash the Channel 9 times.

8. Finish the exercise by collecting Energy at the navel.

Governor Channel Breathing

WE HAVE BEEN WORKING FOR a number of weeks now raising Chi and Jing Chi up to, and breathing into, various points on the Governor Channel. The Governor Channel (Du Mai) is the primary route of the Microcosmic Orbit. It is the Yang Channel. This week we will conclude our work on this Channel.

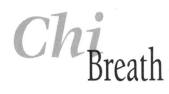

You have learned to open the Governor Channel from the perineum (Hui Yin) all the way up to the Crown Point (Pai Hui). There are still two more points that are necessary to open and work with in order to finish the Governor Channel and move into the Functional Channel and complete the Microcosmic Orbit. Luckily you are all long familiar with both of these points. They are the Third Eye Point (Yin Tang) at the top of the bridge of the nose between the two eyebrows, and the Yen Chong, the point below the center of the nose just above the upper lip. You learned to massage these two points in Week One, Taoist Self-Massage Rejuvenation.

This week you are going to learn to breathe into seven different points on the Governor Channel. This technique is similar to the Reverse Breathing techniques you have been working with since Week Nine. It is just a little more complicated. Instead of taking one continuous reverse inhalation, you will instead take seven small reverse sips of air. With each sip of air you will contract the lower abdomen and push the anus toward a point on the Governor Channel beginning with the coccyx, then the Ming Men, Chi Chung, Jade

Pillow, Crown Point, Third Eye and finally the Yen Chong which is actually in the upper gums above the two front teeth. You will then relax, reverse direction and mentally lower the Energy back down the Governor Channel to the Ming Men and exhale as you pour it into the Tan Tien.

This is a very invigorating breathing exercise. It is a step beyond anything you've learned up to now. Be aware of any strain or tightness as you do it. Be sure not to overdo it! This is a great technique for opening the Governor Channel. As you can see, many of the exercises overlap and work together with each other. You've actually been learning at least three methods for opening the Governor Channel and ultimately the Microcosmic Orbit:

1. This week using breath;
2. Using Jing Chi in Testicle/Ovarian Breathing; and
3. Using the mind in the Microcosmic Orbit exercises.

I've maintained the three-pronged approach of regulating the Breath, Body and Mind (Chi, Jing and Shen), even if I haven't always been telling you that this is what I was doing.

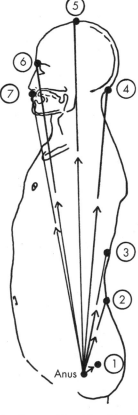

1 – Coccyx   2 – Ming Men
3 – Chi Chung   4 – Jade Pillow
5 – Crown Point   6 – Third Eye
7 – Yen Chong

1. Raise the tip of your tongue to the roof of your mouth, just behind your front teeth. Do a few Abdominal Breaths to begin, then exhale and contract the lower abdomen.

2. Inhale a sip of air, contract the lower abdomen and push your anus toward the coccyx. Mentally direct Chi into the sacral hiatus and sacrum.

3. Take a second sip of air, contract the lower abdomen and push your anus toward the Ming Men Point on your spine opposite the navel. Mentally direct Chi to this point.

4. Take a third sip of air, contract the lower abdomen and push your anus toward the Chi Chung (T-11) Point in your middle back. Mentally direct Chi to this point.

5. Take a fourth sip of air, contract the lower abdomen and push your anus toward the Jade Pillow at the base of the skull. Mentally direct Chi to this point.

6. Take a fifth sip of air, contract the lower abdomen and push your anus toward the

Crown Point at the midpoint of the top of the skull. Mentally direct Chi to this point.

7. Take a sixth sip of air, contract the lower abdomen and push your anus toward the Third Eye Point at the point between the two eyebrows. Mentally direct Chi to this point.

8. Take a seventh sip of air, contract the lower abdomen and push your anus toward the Yen Chong Point on your upper gums just below the midpoint of your nostrils. Mentally direct Chi to this point.

9. Pause for a moment, then relax and mentally direct the Chi back over your head and down your spine to the Ming Men Point. When you reach this point, begin to exhale and pour the Chi into your Tan Tien. Feel the Sea of Chi expanding.

10. Repeat at least 3 times initially and work your way up to nine or more.

If you find yourself running out of breath as you raise the Chi up the Governor Channel, take smaller sips of air or move up the Governor Channel more quickly. If you don't initially feel all the points as you breathe toward them, just imagine that you do (this might be true of the two new points, Third Eye and Yen Chong, we are working with this week). With a little practice you should have no difficulty.

Taoist Self-Massage Rejuvenation: Hitting to Detoxify the Arms

HITTING AND SLAPPING THE ARMS have the same beneficial effects of removing toxins, increasing blood circulation, stimulating the bone marrow, softening and loosening up the muscles and tendons and clearing blockages from the Energy Channels as all the other hitting and slapping techniques you've learned so far.

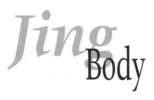

We will hit and slap four different lines in each arm: middle line, thumb line, back line and pinkie line. As in Hitting the Legs Self-Massage, first you slap down the arm with an open palm and then reverse and hit back up the arm with a loosely held fist.

1. Rub your hands together until hot. Begin with the left arm.

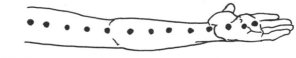

Middle Line

2. The Middle Line: Raise your left arm slightly above shoulder level. Your palm is open, facing upward and your fingers are extended forward. Bring your open right palm to the left side of your neck. Begin slapping down the side of the neck, toward the shoulder, down the biceps, the inside of the elbow, the middle of the forearm, over the wrist to the middle finger. Reverse and hit with the fist, back to the side of your neck.

3. The Thumb Line: Raise your left arm slightly above shoulder level. Your left hand is open but this time the thumb faces upward so that your palm is vertical and facing toward the right side of your body. With your right hand, slap down from the side of your neck, over the shoulder and down the outside of the arm to the base of the thumb. Reverse and hit back up the arm to the side of the neck with a loosely held fist.

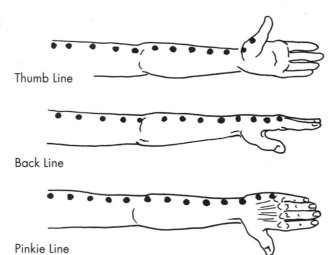

Thumb Line

Back Line

Pinkie Line

4. The Back Line: Keep the left arm raised slightly above the shoulder. Your open palm faces downward toward the ground. Slap with the right hand from the side of your neck down to the back of your middle finger. Reverse and hit upward with a loosely held fist to the side of the neck.

5. The Pinkie Line: Lower your left arm in front of you. Turn your palm outward so it is pointing to your left side. Your pinkie is on top and your thumb points toward the ground. Keep your fingers together (not splayed apart). Again hit with your open right hand from the side of your neck, over your shoulder and down your left arm to the pinkie finger. Reverse and hit upwards with a lightly held fist up to the side of your neck.

6. Repeat steps 2 through 5 on your right arm. Slap and hit with your left hand.

Tao In: Part Three

The Tao In exercises you've learned up to now are the best exercises I know to strengthen the lower back and psoas muscles. This is important to the practice for a number of reasons. For one, the lower back is often the weakest part of the body. Strengthening this region permits us to activate the sacral pump and sacrum. The sacral pump moves inward toward the front of the body at the tail end of the lower back. The top portion of the sacrum moves outward, toward the back, in the region of the Ming Men behind the navel. This pumping action of the lower portion of the spine actually pumps the spinal fluid up the backbone. It stretches the spine and helps break up Energy blockages. It allows both Chi and Jing Chi to flow smoothly up the spine. It is crucial for the sexual practices. When properly activated it helps you to root into the ground and use the Earth Energy to support you. Overall it strengthens the structure of the body and helps you to stand straighter and walk easier.

This week I will finish the psoas set with one final exercise known as the Bow. We will then continue with three stretching exercises that work the whole body.

It is important to remember that the Chi Kung exercises in this book, the Eight Pieces of Brocade, the Muscle-Tendon Change and currently Tao In, are designed to limber you up, strengthen you, keep you healthy and improve the flow of Vital Energy throughout your body. They were not necessarily designed to give you a body beautiful. Some of the best practitioners I've ever met didn't look like martial artists or aerobic instructors at all. They looked very ordinary, sometimes they even looked weak or flabby. But underlying this were the secrets of Internal Power that they possessed. You have been learning many of those secrets in this book. Perineum Power, the sacral and cranial pump, Reverse Breathing, swallowing saliva, protecting the aura and the Microcosmic Orbit—all of these are important to Internal Power. This practice known as Nei Kung was often considered to be the highest form of martial arts.

It is the knowledge of Internal Power, Nei Kung, that transforms the physical exercises or Wei Kung, such as Tao In and Yi Chin Ching, into something more than simple calisthenics. Knowing how to direct Chi with your mind, breath and Perineum Power turns these exercises into physical expressions of Internal Power.

I said earlier that doing Tai Chi Chuan is just an elegant dance unless you know correct breathing and control of the flow of Chi. I was really talking about the knowledge of Internal Power. This is what it's all about.

Tao In #9: The Bow

1. Lie flat on your back with your legs together, stretched out straight and your arms by your sides.

2. Inhale an Abdominal Breath and remain relaxed.

3. Exhale slowly and raise your legs and feet off the ground.

4. Simultaneously raise your torso from the waist. Lift your arms and stretch your fingertips toward your toes. Try to keep your neck as straight as possible.

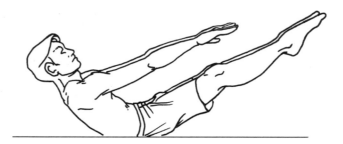

5. Your body looks V-shaped as you simultaneously lift the legs and torso. Activate the Sacral Pump and keep the lower back in contact with the ground as you raise up both the legs and torso.

6. It is not necessary that you actually touch your toes, just reach for them and raise up as far as you can as you slowly exhale. As you complete the exhalation you can bend the head and neck forward to get the maximum stretch.

7. Sink back to the floor, relax and inhale.

8. Repeat 3 or more times if you can.

Tao In #10: The Reverse Bow

1. Lie on your stomach. Your arms are stretched out in front of you and your legs are straight behind you.

2. Inhale an Abdominal Breath and remain relaxed.

3. Exhale slowly and simultaneously raise up your legs and torso. Arch from your navel which remains in contact with the floor so that your body looks like a V.

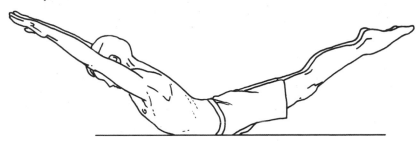

4. Activate your Cranial Pump, pulling your chin in, and pushing the back of the head backward and upward, to keep your neck straight.

5. Your arms are lifted off the ground above the level of your shoulders. Extend and stretch the fingers straight forward.

6. Stretch your toes straight back.

7. Lower your body, relax and inhale.

8. Repeat 3 or more times if you can.

Tao In #11: Lying Stretch

1. Lie flat on your back. Your arms are stretched out on the ground behind your head. Your feet are stretched out straight forward on the ground.

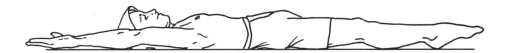

2. Inhale an Abdominal Breath and relax.

3. Exhale slowly and activate the Sacral Pump to flatten your lower back to the ground and activate the Cranial Pump to push the back of your neck as close to the ground as possible.

4. Extend and stretch your arms and fingers straight back behind your head. Simultaneously stretch your toes forward. Do not lift your arms or legs off the ground. But keep your lower back in contact with the ground.

5. Relax and inhale.

6. Repeat 3 or more times.

Tao In #12: Lying Toe Pull

1. Lie flat on your back. Your hands are at your sides. Your feet are straight forward on the ground with your toes pointing upward. Raise the tip of your tongue to the roof of your mouth.

2. Inhale an Abdominal Breath and remain relaxed.

3. Exhale and activate the Sacral and Cranial Pumps and flatten your back and neck into the ground.

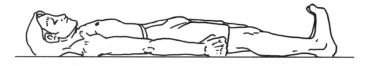

4. Exhale slowly. Without otherwise moving your legs, pull your toes toward your head.

5. Simultaneously tighten your hands into fists and push the middle finger of each hand into the center of the palm.

6. Relax and inhale.

7. Repeat 3 or more times.

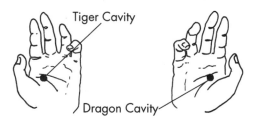

Pressing into the center of the palm with the middle finger activates the Dragon Cavity in the right hand and the Tiger Cavity in the left. Both of these cavities are linked to the heart (pericardium) and lower abdomen. These are also important points for controlling sexual desire and controlling leakage of Jing Chi.

Sexual Kung Fu: Scrotal and Ovarian Compression

With Scrotal and Ovarian Compression, also known as Compression Breathing, we move on to a completely new Sexual Kung Fu technique and I finally get a chance to teach you about swallowing the breath.

Swallowing the breath is essentially similar to swallowing saliva except that the mouth is filled with air, and the air is swallowed hard, with a gulping sound. There are various uses in Taoist Yoga for this technique. A basic use is to force more air into the lungs when they seem already packed. It is also an excellent technique for loosening up a tight, constricted throat. Try it. On another level altogether, swallowing air or saliva at the moment of impact of a punch or kick was among the most secret techniques of Taoist martial artists. It added tremendous power when coordinated with the strike. On still another level, swallowing air was the primary practice of advanced Tao Masters who existed on little else but air itself. These were the Breatharians. Many of their practices are documented and recorded in the Taoist Canon. The basic practice consists of swallowing air as I described above. If done sufficiently, this seems to inhibit the appetite. Although the exact mechanism is not known, it seems that oxygen was somehow able to pass right through the walls of the lower abdomen. The Breatharians after years of practice were able to subsist on little else but air alone. Eventually all their bodily functions would slow down to the point where their body seemed to be in a state of suspended animation. Having also developed the Spirit Body, their consciousness could exit and enter their body at will. Supposedly these Taoist adepts could survive in this state for extraordinarily long periods of time, which to us would seem to be many lifetimes. Personally I have never met one and don't know anyone who has. But based on translations of authentic Taoist texts, I'm reasonably certain that they did exist once, in mountainous retreats in ancient China.

Scrotal/Ovarian Compression provides us with yet another use for Swallowing the Breath. The breath is swallowed and compressed and moved down the body in the shape of a ball which is eventually pushed or compressed into the scrotum or ovaries resulting in a tremendous boost of Sexual Energy. Compression Breathing greatly magnifies the benefits of both Testicle and Ovarian Breathing, which we finished learning last week. For both men and women, with regular practice, it works to relieve conditions of low energy and fatigue. It helps us to learn to direct Energy into and out of the pelvic and sexual region. It is an excellent way to quickly energize your body especially if you're feeling down or weak. It works as a general tonic for the nervous system helping to reduce nervousness and insomnia.

While the exercise is basically identical for men and women, its other benefits differ, depending on your gender.

For men this exercise helps to prevent premature ejaculation and the loss of semen in our sleep from wet dreams. It strengthens the muscles of the entire sexual region. Its practice helps to calm down overexcited sexual desires. Most importantly it compresses Chi, drawn out of the air we breathe, into the testicles to strengthen our Jing Chi.

For women some of the benefits are similar and some are quite different. It increases the strength of the vaginal muscles as well as the cervix and ovaries. But whereas Scrotal Compression helps men to tame their sexuality, Ovarian Compression has the opposite effect on women. By compressing Chi into the ovaries and vagina, this area is warmed up, creating more Yang Jing Chi. When the sexual organs are warm, women are more easily aroused and it is easier to reach orgasm. Remember, women do not lose Jing from orgasm, only men do.

As I said, the exercise itself is basically identical for men and women, up to the final steps anyway. I'll begin with the first few steps generically then finish with separate instructions for men and women.

This exercise can be done sitting, standing or lying down. I will describe the standing position. Wear loose-fitting clothing. Men should wear underwear that allows the testicles to hang freely.

1. Stand with feet facing forward, shoulder width apart. Raise the tip of your tongue to the upper palate.

2. Breathe a Reverse Breath slowly through the nose. Inhale completely until the air fills the throat and you cannot inhale any more.

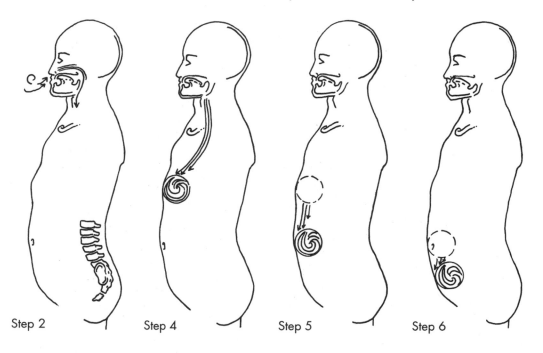

Step 2   Step 4   Step 5   Step 6

3. Swallow the air with a gulping sound.

4. Push the air down to the solar plexus. Push out on the solar plexus and feel/imagine the air becoming compressed and ball shaped. Don't use a lot of force when you push out.

5. Press or roll the ball of air down to the navel. Push out at the navel level.

6. Press or roll the ball down to the lower abdomen, and gently push it outward.

Men:

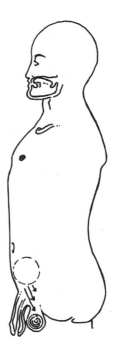

7. Press or roll the ball of air down to the scrotum (the sac containing the testicles), by contracting the abdominal muscles downward like a slow wave.

8. Keep the tongue raised to the roof of the mouth and forcibly push and compress the ball of air into the scrotum for as long as you can. You should be able to do this for at least 10 seconds. Work up to a minute or more. You hold your breath as you do this.

9. Simultaneously squeeze the perineum and anus to prevent loss of Energy.

10. Exhale and relax completely.

11. Do a few short, rapid Abdominal Breaths (Bellows Breathing). Then return to normal breathing.

12. Repeat a minimum of 3 times per session and increase this number as you are able.

13. Conclude the exercise by rotating the waist as in the Screwing the Hips exercise from Week Eight, Taoist Self-Massage Rejuvenation.

Women:

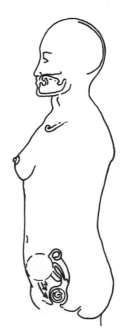

7. Contract the abdominal muscles in a wave-like motion to push the ball of air down to the ovaries where it spreads out to both sides of the body.

8. Tightly squeeze the inner and outer lips of the vagina as well as your perineum and anus.

9. Forcibly push and compress the air into your ovaries for a minimum of 10 seconds. Try to work up to one minute. You are holding your breath as you do this.

10. As you compress the air downward, push into your vagina, which will feel as if it is expanding.

11. Exhale and relax completely.

12. Do a few short, rapid Abdominal Breaths (Bellows Breathing). Then return to normal breathing.

13. Repeat a minimum of 3 times per session and increase this number as you are able.

14. Conclude the exercise by rotating the waist as in the Screwing the Hips exercise from Week Eight, Taoist Self-Massage Rejuvenation.

There may be a tendency to pass gas when you first start to practice. This is another reason the anus and perineum are squeezed tightly during the compression. Once you get the hang of this exercise, this should no longer be a problem.

Compression Breathing is a powerful technique. You should start to feel its effects almost immediately. You can do this exercise by itself or before doing Testicle/Ovarian Breathing. Do a few rounds of Scrotal/Ovarian Compression and then do the Testicle/Ovarian Breathing. With a little practice you should feel the Jing Chi literally shoot up your spine and into your head. Women, remember to lower this hot Energy down to the Tan Tien. Men can do this, too, to prevent any build-up of pressure in the skull.

The Microcosmic Orbit: Part Five

Shen
Mind

WE ARE NEARING THE COMPLETION of the Microcosmic Orbit. Because of the nature of what I am teaching, I had to construct this book to move at a moderate, balanced pace. A lot of thought has gone into how to coordinate each week's material so that it is logical, coherent, builds upon itself, and ultimately holds together. I realize that what I am doing here has never been done before and that is to create a week-by-week approach to accomplish the 100 Days of Practice necessary to build a solid foundation in Taoist Yoga. This 100 days is not a number I chose at random. The 100 Days is mentioned in *The Secret of the Golden Flower* as well as in almost all authentic Taoist texts. Mantak Chia gives his new students who have studied the Microcosmic Orbit with him a practice guide for 100 Days of Practice. His students have already learned the Microcosmic Orbit at the start of their 100 days. As a result, their practice is very different in many ways from what you've learned here. If I taught you the Microcosmic Orbit at the start of this book, most of you would probably have understood what I was talking about intellectually, but few of you would have been able to control and direct the Chi through the various points on the Orbit. I hope that the methodical step-by-step approach I have used has led you to not only understand what I write about, but to experience it as well.

You have been working on this material for almost three months now. Hopefully you are reaping some of the benefits of Chi Kung and Taoist Yoga. In these Regulating the Mind exercises you have been learning true Third Treasure methods of Taoist meditation. I am sure that many of you can now feel the warm Chi current moving through the Energy Channels. We have come a long way in these three months.

One of the real secrets of the Golden Flower is the circulation of the light. In some of the practices you should have experienced this light. In Week Seven I introduced you to the golden light in the back line of the Inner Smile. This light is associated with Yang Energy and the Sun. It has a Yin counterpart and often appears as soft moonlight. This light first manifests just in front of or behind the point referred to as the Third Eye, also called the Mid-Eye Point, the Yin Tang, Tsu Chiao, Cavity of Original Spirit or Heavenly Heart. The actual location of the point is three inches directly behind the midpoint between the eyebrows. It is the pituitary gland. The Taoists called this the Square Inch Field or Central Castle. We have been working in this area since Week Two. It is not necessary to direct your mind three inches inside the brain, just focusing on the Third Eye Point is sufficient and the light should shine inward of its own accord. This is also the Backward Flowing Method. If the light appears as a perfectly round and white or silvery moonlike object, this is a sure sign of progress.

The pituitary gland is part of the Crystal Palace, as is the pineal gland. It is about the size of a pea and is one of the most important endocrine glands in the body, producing a wide range of hormones that trigger and control such varied functions as stimulating thyroid activity to the secretion of breast milk and manufacture of testosterone. To the Taoists it was the home of the Spirit. The Spirit is the light. When the light shines in front of or behind the Yin Tang like the Moon, this is a sure sign that the Master, the Original Mind, is being restored to its rightful place as the silent ruler of your mind.

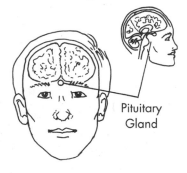

Pituitary Gland

If you didn't understand any of the above, just keep on with the practice; in time you will understand. For those of you who did comprehend it, you have surely made great progress in the practice of the Tao.

When the Third Eye Point is open, you experience wisdom. When it is closed down you are indecisive and incapable of making decisions.

The final point on the Governor Channel is the Palate Point that I have told you to raise the tip of your tongue to so many times in this book. We have done most of our work on the Wind Point directly behind the front teeth. Farther back on the hard palate is the Fire Point. This point is useful in drawing hot Yang energy from the brain. If you raise your tongue and curl it backwards, your tongue will touch the soft palate also known as the Water Point or Heavenly 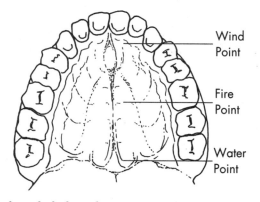 Pool (Hsuan Ying). This point lies directly below the pituitary gland. This is a useful point when circulating Sexual Energy. When you raise your tongue to connect the Functional Channel to the Governor Channel, experiment with where it feels most comfortable and the Chi seems to flow most easily.

This week we will actually move into the Functional Channel as we lower the Chi through the raised tip of the tongue, down through the tongue to the Throat Point just above the V-like notch at the front base of the neck. I have already discussed many of the properties of this point in Week Six, Taoist Self-Massage Rejuvenation. It is the seat of speech and communications. It is also intimately related with Taoist Dream Yoga which is called lucid dreaming in the West. Focus on this point as you go to sleep and try to maintain your consciousness as you cross the boundary between the waking and dream states.

The Throat Point is one of the weakest and most difficult to protect of all the points in the body. Massage and circulating Chi through it in the Microcosmic Orbit are the best ways to protect it. The Taoists believed that a weak Throat Point allowed you to be easily controlled by others and was the place where evil spirits could enter the body. When the Throat Point is open, you are more eloquent. When it is closed down, you feel an unwillingness to change.

1. Begin by focusing on the tip of the nose. Once you feel calm and centered raise your point of concentration to the Third Eye Point. Smile into your eyes then do as much of the Inner Smile as you have time for. This can vary each time you practice, but it should under no circumstances be ignored.

2. Return your concentration to the Third Eye Point. Your eyelids should be lowered but not completely closed. Let your eyesight turn around as if you were looking inward. Make saliva, raise your tongue to the roof of your mouth, and swallow with a gulping sound. Guide the Energy with your inner eyes as it descends to your Tan Tien so that your eyes are looking down and inside of you. From now on you will use your inner eyesight as well as your mind to guide the Chi to each point on the Orbit.

3. Do Bellows Breathing to Warm the Stove. Exhale and lower the Chi to the Sperm/Ovarian Palace. Let your inner eyesight guide the Chi. Inhale an Abdominal Breath then exhale and lower the Chi to your perineum as you guide it down with your inner eyesight.

4. Inhale a Reverse Breath, pull up on the perineum, anus and coccyx (Perineum Power) and guide the Chi with your inner eyesight through the sacral hiatus and up to the Ming Men. It is as if your eyes could turn upward and inward from the perineum point and see the Chi go up the spine. Physically this is impossible, but your inner eyes can do it. Exhale and lower the Chi back to your perineum.

5. In the same manner raise the Chi to the Chi Chung (T-11), Jade Pillow and Crown Points.

6. Exhale and lower the Chi all the way down the Governor Channel to your perineum. Return your concentration and inner eyesight to the perineum. Inhale a Reverse Breath, use Perineum Power and raise the Chi all the way up the Governor Channel to your Crown Point. Guide the Chi with your inner eyesight, which is now looking inward and upward to the Crown Point.

7. Exhale and guide the Chi forward and downward to the Third Eye Point. Inhale and raise it back to the Crown Point. Wash the Channel 6 times. Be sure to maintain your inner eyesight.

8. Exhale and guide the Chi back to the Third Eye (Pituitary) Point. Maintain your concentration on this point for a minute or more.

9. Inhale and guide the Chi back to the Crown Point. Exhale and guide the Chi down the Governor Channel to your perineum.

10. Inhale a Reverse Breath. Use Perineum Power and guide the Chi all the way up the Governor Channel, past the Crown Point to the Third Eye Point.

11. Exhale and guide the Chi down through the nose to the Palate Point in the roof of your mouth. Wash the Channel from the Palate to the Third Eye Point 6 times.

12. Exhale and guide the Chi back to the Palate Point. Maintain your concentration on this point for a minute or more.

13. Inhale and guide the Chi back to the Crown Point. Exhale and guide the Chi down the Governor Channel to your perineum.

14. Inhale a Reverse Breath. Use Perineum Power and guide the Chi all the way up the Governor Channel, past the Crown Point and Third Eye Point to your Palate Point.

15. Exhale and guide the Chi with your inner eyesight into the tip of your raised tongue, through your tongue, down to the Throat Center at the base of the throat.

16. Wash the Channel from Throat to Palate Point 6 times.

17. Exhale and guide the Chi back to the Throat Center. Maintain your concentration here for a minute or more.

18. Inhale an Abdominal Breath, exhale and guide the Chi down the Functional Channel to the Tan Tien behind and slightly below your navel.

19. Collect the Energy. Rub your hands together until hot and massage your face and eyes.

YOU'VE REACHED THE PENULTIMATE WEEK of these 100 Days of Practice. If you've come this far, you will no doubt complete the practice. You are sure to be experiencing positive results like feeling stronger and healthier, calmer and more relaxed. Sexually, you should be feeling more secure and self-confident.

You may have also experienced new and unusual states of mind while doing the Regulating the Mind exercises. Sometimes you might experience visions of snow falling from the sky, or of trees standing in rows. You might think you hear indistinct voices or music in the distance when nobody is there. Treat any unusual experience with indifference. Do not let yourself get emotionally involved in it. Do not be moved if it happens, do not be moved if it does not happen. These are a few examples of *confirmatory experiences*. For each of us, what we experience can be completely different, or not happen at all. Pay it no mind. This is the true Taoist attitude. Just know that they are signs of progress.

This week we complete the Microcosmic Orbit. We begin by fully opening the Functional Channel. You will also learn to raise aroused Sexual Energy. I told you earlier in this book that the best was yet to come. Well, here it is.

Functional Channel Breathing

YOU ARE ALREADY FAMILIAR WITH all the points on the Functional Channel. All we have to do this week is connect them. The Functional Channel runs up, or down, the front of the body from the perineum to the tip of your tongue.

*Chi*Breath

In this week's exercise you will breathe into six points on the Functional Channel: the Sperm/Ovarian Palace, the navel, the solar plexus, the heart center in the middle of the sternum (the thymus gland), the throat center and the tip of the tongue. You will use Abdominal Breathing for this exercise, not Reverse Breathing as we have in the past few weeks' Regulating the Breath exercises.

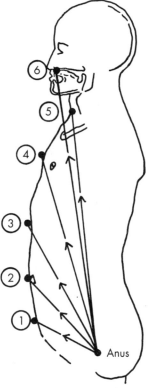

1 – Sperm/Ovarian Palace
2 – Navel Point   3 – Solar Plexus
4 – Heart Point   5 – Throat Point
6 – Tip of Raised Tongue

1. Raise the tip of your tongue to the roof of your mouth, just behind your teeth (the Wind Point). Begin by inhaling an Abdominal Breath. However, do not completely expand the lower abdomen. Leave room to take 6 small sips of air as you move up the Functional Channel.

2. Inhale a sip of air, slightly expand the lower abdomen and push your anus toward the Sperm/Ovarian Palace. Mentally direct Chi toward this point.

3. Take a second sip of air, slightly expand your lower abdomen and push your anus toward your navel. Mentally direct Chi to this point.

4. Take a third sip of air, slightly expand your lower abdomen and push your anus toward your solar plexus. Mentally direct Chi to this point.

5. Take a fourth sip of air, slightly expand your lower abdomen and push your anus toward the Heart Point in the middle of your sternum (breastbone). This is also the location of your thymus gland. Mentally direct Chi to this point.

6. Take a fifth sip of air, slightly expand your lower abdomen and push your anus toward the Throat Point at the bottom of your throat. Mentally direct Chi to this point.

7. Take a sixth sip of air, slightly expand your lower abdomen and push your anus toward the tip of your raised tongue. Push your tongue against the upper palate Wind Point. Mentally direct Chi to this point.

8. Pause for a moment, then relax and mentally direct the Chi back down the Functional Channel to your navel. When you reach this point, begin to exhale and pour the Chi into your Tan Tien.

9. Repeat at least 3 times initially and work your way up to 9 or more.

Taoist Self-Massage Rejuvenation: Massaging the Sternum

THE STERNUM OR BREASTBONE IS in the center of your chest between the ribs. Massaging the sternum helps to open your Heart Center which we will be working with in this week's Regulating the Mind exercise. It also helps to activate the thymus gland which lies close to the top of the sternum. This gland is the most important gland for Taoist rejuvenation. It plays a crucial role in the body's immune system. As we age, it tends to shrink considerably in size. Massaging the sternum along with opening the Microcosmic Orbit, as well as many other of the exercises you've learned in this book, help to revitalize and grow the thymus gland.

Jing Body

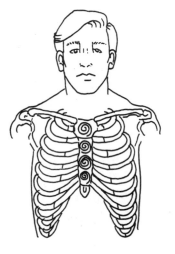

The sternum massage also helps to relieve shortness of breath, release negative emotions and stimulates the flow of lymph.

1. Use the index finger knuckle or middle finger knuckle.

2. Massage in small circles from the top to the bottom of your sternum.

3. If you find any painful spots, spend more time there but be careful not to overdo it at first. The sternum can become sore afterwards.

Massaging the Hands

You have been massaging your hands since the very beginning of these 100 Days of Practice. Each time you rub your hands together until they are warm or hot you are stimulating the six Energy Channels in each hand. I'd like to give you a more efficient method for Warming the Hands.

Warming the Hands

1. Inhale a Reverse Breath.

2. Contract the entire perineum area including the sexual organs.

3. Hold your breath and mentally direct Chi to your hands and fingertips.

4. Rub your hands together until hot.

5. Repeat whenever your hands cool down during any of the Self-Massage exercises.

Massaging the Dragon and Tiger Cavities

As you learned in last week's Tao In #12, Lying Down and Pulling the Toes, the Dragon Cavity of the right hand and the Tiger Cavity of the left are found at the point where the tip of the middle finger meets the palm when you make a fist. Massaging here will break up Energy blockages and stimulate the pericardium which is the fascia surrounding the heart, the heart itself and the lower abdomen.

1. Warm your hands as above.

2. Use the thumb of the left hand to massage the Dragon Cavity in the right hand.

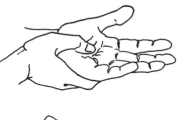

3. Use the thumb of the right hand to massage the Tiger Cavity of the left hand.

4. Massage with a circular motion.

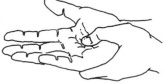

Massaging the Hegu

The Hegu point is located in the fleshy area between your thumb and your index finger. It is generally found closer to the index finger, but you must massage around the area until you find the most painful point. That's the Hegu.

In most of us it's easy to find because when you massage it, it hurts like hell. The Hegu is also known as the Large Intestine Point and massaging here will stimulate the Channel for the large intestines. In traditional Chinese medicine the Hegu massage was indicated for headache, toothache, sore throats, dizziness, insomnia and eye disorders.

1. Warm your hands.

2. Press the thumb of the right hand into the Hegu point on the outer part of the left hand. Support the inside of the left hand with the index finger of the right hand.

3. Massage in a circular motion until the pain dissolves or you can't take it anymore.

4. Reverse hands and massage.

Hegu

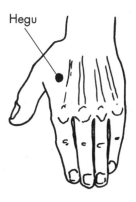

Dry Washing

This is a technique that is practiced throughout China to massage the hands and prevent arthritis.

1. Place your right palm over the back of your left hand. The fingers of your right hand reach over the pinkie side of the left hand, resting in the middle of the left palm.

2. Grasp the left hand tightly in the right hand and pull the hands apart.

3. Repeat a few times, then switch hands.

Tao In: Part Four

This week you'll practice a variety of four different types of Tao In exercises. These positions are especially useful for the upper back and shoulders. They are a little more complex to describe than most of the others you've learned. If you follow the directions carefully, you should have no problem. I learned all the Tao In exercises in this book from Master Mantak Chia. Most of them have never been described in book form before.

Tao In #13: Bend to Knee and Raise the Shoulder

This is a marvelous exercise for stretching the tendons of the body. You stretch the arms, legs, spine, back and shoulders. Pay special attention to the final stretch, as you slowly turn the back muscles and raise the shoulder. First turn from the lower back, then turn the middle back muscles, finally turn the upper back muscles. Do them one section at a time, not simultaneously.

1. Sit on the ground with your left leg stretched out in front of you.

2. Your right leg is on the ground with your knee bent and your right foot tucked into your groin against the top of your left thigh. Inhale an Abdominal Breath.

3. Begin exhaling slowly and reach forward and grasp the raised toes of your left foot with your left hand. If you cannot bend this far, try to grasp your left ankle. Your right hand rests on your right knee.

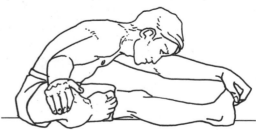

4. Slowly bend your left elbow to your left knee. Lower your head slowly toward your left knee. Starting with your lower back, feel the vertebra open one by one.

5. When you get your head as close to your left knee as you can, push your right hand against your right knee and straighten your right arm. This will push your right shoulder upward and back.

6. Slowly turn your trunk to the right as you push your right hand against your right knee and straighten your right arm. Turn first from the lower back muscles.

7. Next turn to the right a little more as you move from the middle back muscles.

8. Finally turn the upper back muscles to the right, raising and pushing back your right shoulder as far as possible. Your head will turn to the right as your shoulder moves upward and back. *Don't use your neck muscles to turn it.*

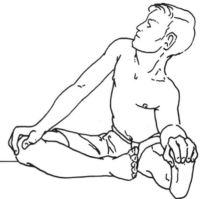

9. Relax, do a total of 3 times and then reverse sides.

Try to get into the habit of turning your shoulders when you want to turn your head. This results in much less tension on the muscles and tendons in the neck. This exercise and the following one are designed to open and loosen up those tight shoulders.

Tao In #14: Push and Pull the Leg

This is another three-part exercise. It is fairly simple and provides a great tendon and muscle stretch for the whole body, but especially the upper back and shoulders. The idea here is to keep one hand on your outstretched leg, just above the knee. This is your pushing hand. In each of the three positions, with one arm you push on your leg and straighten your arm, just as in the previous exercise. With the other arm, you bend forward and turn the torso and grab and hold on to the same outstretched leg in three separate positions:

1. On the upper calf, just below the knee;

2. At mid-calf, halfway between the knee and the ankle; and

3. The foot.

This is the pulling position. You pull from any of the three positions as you push with the other hand above the knee.

Start in the same position as Tao In #13.

Part A:

1. Sit on the ground with your left leg stretched out in front of you.

2. Your right leg is bent at the knee with your right foot tucked into your groin against the top of your left thigh. Inhale an Abdominal Breath.

3. Place your left hand on your thigh, just above your knee.

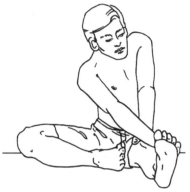

4. Bend forward and reach across your body with your right arm and grab the top of your left calf, just below the knee, with your right hand.

5. Begin to exhale slowly. Pull against your left calf with your right arm.

6. Simultaneously push against your left leg, just above your knee, with your left hand. Push until your left arm is straight.

7. As you simultaneously push and pull, your body turns to the left, your right shoulder sinks and your left shoulder is pushed upward. Stretch as far as you can.

8. Exhale and relax.

Part B:

1. Place your right hand on the midpoint of the left calf, between your knee and your ankle. Except for this change and the fact that you have to bend forward more, repeat the exercise as in Part A.

Part C:

1. Place your right hand across the sole of your left foot. If you cannot bend and reach this far, then just grab your left ankle. Repeat the exercise as in Part A.

2. Repeat with right leg stretched forward and left foot bent into the groin. Do all 3 positions.

Tao In #15: Pushing Mountains

Pushing Mountains can be done standing or sitting. It is a simple exercise, but again pay attention to the details. This one is excellent for stretching and opening the vertebra of the upper back. We push both raised hands out to the side of our body as we turn our head in the opposite direction.

1. Start with your arms at your sides. Bend your right arm at the elbow and bring your right hand up next to your right shoulder, open palm facing right, away from your body. Your elbow remains sunk down, close to but not touching the side of your body.

2. Again bending at the elbow, raise and bring your left hand across your body to your right shoulder. Your open left palm also faces right. Your elbow remains bent and close to your body on the left side.

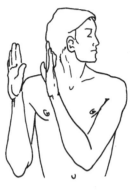

3. Turn your head to the left (the opposite direction from your open palms).

4. Inhale and remain relaxed.

5. Exhale slowly and squeeze your hands and arms as you learned in the Muscle-Tendon Change Classic. Simultaneously push both hands to the right side as you squeeze. Your arms don't actually move that much as you both squeeze and push at the same time. Imagine that you are pushing mountains aside with your Internal Power.

6. Turn your head as far to the left as you can as you push and squeeze with your arms and hands.

7. Inhale and relax your neck and sink your elbows in.

8. Repeat 3 times.

9. Reverse sides and push and squeeze with your hands and arms toward the left side, as you turn your head to the right. Repeat 3 times.

Tao In #16: Arm Tendon Twist

This exercise is especially useful for the tendons of the forearms and hands as well as the shoulder and side of the neck. It can be done standing or sitting.

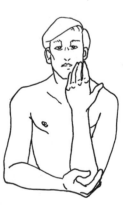

1. Inhale and bend the elbow of your left arm in front of your body, so that your elbow points downward at about the level of your solar plexus. Your left arm and hand are raised, with your left palm facing you, in front of your face.

2. With your right hand, cup your left elbow and pull it into the middle of your body. Hold the left elbow in place, close to your solar plexus for the remainder of the exercise.

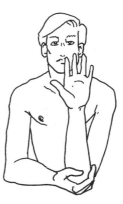

3. Exhale slowly and starting at your left wrist, squeeze your raised left hand and forearm.

4. As you squeeze, use the tendons of the left forearm to turn your left palm outward, away from your face.

5. Relax and repeat a few times, then reverse hands.

Sexual Kung Fu: The Power Lock Exercise

If we hadn't taken five weeks to methodically learn Testicle/Ovarian Breathing, we would have to spend at least an equal amount of time learning the Power Lock Exercise. Fortunately, taking into account everything that you have already learned, you should be able to grasp the essentials of the Power Lock in just a week.

In this exercise, both men and women learn to draw aroused Sexual Energy up the spine to the brain. The route is identical to Testicle/Ovarian Breathing.

This is a self-cultivation exercise which means that no partner is required. You have to arouse the Jing Chi yourself. For men this requires using masturbation to arouse yourself to the point just before orgasm. You must stop before you reach "the point of no return." Women should first massage their breasts as described in Week Three. This should start feelings of arousal. Direct these sexual feelings down to your ovaries and vagina. Then use masturbation to arouse yourself even more. When you feel fully aroused or reach orgasm, you can begin doing the Orgasmic Upward Draw. Women do not lose Jing during orgasm so there is no problem with raising actual orgasmic energy. However, this might be a little too powerful at first, so it is best to begin doing the exercise before you reach orgasm and keep practicing until you feel ready.

In a reversal from the method used in Testicle Breathing, the aroused Sexual Energy brought up by men is hot Yang Jing Chi and cannot be left in the head. It must be brought down to the Tan Tien or circulated in the Microcosmic Orbit which you will learn to complete this week. For women the opposite is true: the aroused Sexual Energy is cool Yin Jing Chi and this can be left in the head, brought down to the Tan Tien or circulated in the Microcosmic Orbit.

The Power Lock exercises strengthen the spine, and bring powerful rejuvenating Energy to the brain. It also begins the process of transforming our

Third Treasure, Shen, from mental energy into spiritual energy, the basis for more advanced practices than you will learn in these 100 Days of Practice.

The Big Draw for Men

The Big Draw helps you to control the outward flow of semen. The Sexual Energy is instead pushed backward and up the spine to the head. Not the semen, just the Essence of the Sexual Energy.

This is a powerful exercise. It is really necessary to practice this exercise so that you will be able to control yourself during Dual Cultivation practices with a female partner. I assure you that this is an exercise you will have fun practicing.

When you actually do the exercise, a lot of things must happen at once. You will already be familiar with most of what I'll describe. When you draw the Sexual Energy up the spine, you will close your eyes and look upward toward the Crown Point. This helps the Jing Chi to rise. You will hold your arms at your sides and tighten and clench both hands into fists. You will also clench your jaw muscles and activate the cranial pump. The remaining details I will set out step-by-step below.

1. Stand with feet shoulder width apart and your knees slightly bent (horse stance). Wear loose-fitting clothing or nothing below the waist.

2. Use your hand to stimulate your penis to erection.

3. Continue masturbating until you are near the point of orgasm. If you pass the "point of no return," quickly use the three-finger method to press on the Million Dollar Point you learned about in Week Three, Seminal Kung Fu for Men, to prevent the loss of semen.

4. Inhale deeply, clench both fists and vigorously press your fists downward, on either side of your thighs.

5. Simultaneously claw your feet into the ground, clench your jaw tight, activate the Cranial Pump and raise the tip of your tongue to the roof of your mouth.

6. Without exhaling, inhale again and draw up the genitals, anus, perineum and urogenital diaphragm, tightly squeezing the penis.

7. Your closed eyes look upward toward your Crown Point and you mentally direct the Jing Chi through the sacral hiatus and up the spine, through the Jade Pillow to the Crown Point. Try to activate the Sacral Pump, but this will be difficult at the beginning because of the powerful nature of the aroused Jing Chi.

8. Hold your breath and remain flexed for a count of 9.

9. Exhale and release.

10. If you still have an erection, repeat the exercise.

11. As you learned in Week Eleven, Testicle and Ovarian Breathing: Part 5, spiral the Jing Chi in your head. But you begin this time with counter-clockwise revolutions (from the front to the left side then to the back and return on the right side). You can do 9, 18 or 36 revolutions counter-clockwise and the same number clockwise.

12. When you are finished spiraling, touch the tip of your tongue to the palate and direct the flow of Chi down the Functional Channel to the Tan Tien or into the Microcosmic Orbit.

The Orgasmic Upward Draw for Women

1. Sit with your feet flat on the floor or stand with feet shoulder width apart and knees slightly bent (horse stance).

2. Begin by massaging your breasts as taught in Week Three, Ovarian Kung Fu for Women. This will give rise to erotic feelings in your breasts, clitoris, and vagina.

3. Focus on your nipples and direct the sexual feelings in the breasts down to your ovaries.

4. Allow the Sexual Energy to expand into the Ovarian Palace and into the genitals.

5. Begin to masturbate. When you are near or in the midst of an orgasm, inhale a deep breath, clench both fists and vigorously press your fists downward on either side of your thighs.

6. Simultaneously claw your feet into the ground, clench your jaw tight, activate your Sacral and Cranial Pumps and raise the tip of your tongue to the roof of your mouth.

7. Without exhaling, inhale again and draw up the genitals, anus, perineum and urogenital diaphragm, tightly squeezing the lips of the vagina.

8. Your closed eyes look up toward the Crown Point and you mentally direct the Jing Chi from the Ovarian Palace to the perineum, through the sacral hiatus and up the spine, through the Jade Pillow to the Crown Point (Pai Hui). Feel yourself leading the Sexual Energy up from the Crown Point.

9. Continue to lead the Jing Chi up your spine to the Crown Point. Inhale a sip of air with each Upward Orgasmic Draw.

10. When your lungs are full, exhale. Then inhale again and continue to draw up the Sexual Energy until the feelings of arousal subside in the genitals.

11. As you learned in Week Eleven, Ovarian Breathing: Part 5, spiral the Jing Chi in your head. But you begin this time with clockwise revolutions (from the front to the right side then to the back and return on the left side). You can do 9, 18 or 36 revolutions clockwise and the same number counter-clockwise.

12. When you are finished spiraling, relax and rest for a while.

13. The cool Yin Jing Chi can be left in the brain or you can let it flow down the Functional Channel to the Tan Tien or into the Microcosmic Orbit.

The Energy you feel in your body after you do this exercise may fill you with feelings of universal love and compassion. The Taoists, again borrowing from the Buddhists, believed that compassion was the highest emotion. It is the quintessence of all the positive emotions.

The Microcosmic Orbit: Part Six

Shen Mind SO THIS WEEK WE FINALLY complete the Microcosmic Orbit. Actually you completed it last week when you brought the Chi down from your Throat Center to your Tan Tien. When you did that, the Orbit was completed. But I didn't guide you through the Heart and Solar Plexus Centers, so that is what we'll do this week.

We've come a long way together since you first started this book. You know things now that you probably never even dreamed of before. The really good part is that it's all yours. You did it for yourself and your greatest possession. You can take it with you wherever you go. Nothing you've learned in this book requires you to use any equipment whatsoever. The Taoist treasures are weightless. They can be transported in your head and carried anywhere over the face of this globe without the need of any excess baggage.

Completion of the Microcosmic Orbit is a major event in your life in terms of your health, longevity, rejuvenation and sexuality. It works on all these levels.

We have spent the past twelve weeks preparing for this and learning to raise enough Energy so that you can feel it and control it. By now you know that you really can feel Energy flow where you direct it. You've been working with this Energy-Chi since Week One. But, although it was easy to get in touch with the Life Force Energy inside your body, it is much more difficult to control its direction and flow. This is what I have attempted to teach you in this book.

By this point you should have no difficulty at all feeling Energy or a warm current flow down from the warm stove in your Tan Tien to the Sperm/Ovarian Palace and then to your perineum. With a reverse inhalation, the Chi flows into the sacrum, past the Ming Men, T-11, Jade Pillow to the Crown Point at the top of your head. An exhalation will send the Chi downward to your Third Eye Point and then to the roof of your mouth and Palate Point, where it passes into the tip of your raised tongue and into the Functional Channel.

I have been using a technique called Washing the Channels to help you open the Orbit. You might find it somewhat tedious, but no other practice I know will allow you to feel the Energy so strongly as you move it from just one point to another. We "scrub" or "wash" the Channel by going back and forth and remove any blockages to the free flow of Energy. So now after weeks of practice you are ready to take the final step and connect the last two points on the Orbit.

What is most important is to use your mind, your inner eyesight and your internal hearing to direct the flow of Chi. It is as if you direct these senses to the spot where you want to control the Chi flow and just lead it from there. When you do this, the Energy follows easily and smoothly.

I've said there are many ways to teach the Microcosmic Orbit. Yun Xiang Tseng, the Chi Kung, Tai Chi and Kung Fu Master from mainland China who now teaches on Long Island, New York, tells me that there are over 350 different ways to teach it in China today. The way I've been teaching you works well if you are learning from a book. The most important thing, though, is to open the Microcosmic Orbit.

The Heart Point on the Microcosmic Orbit isn't really at the heart. Its location is one inch up from the bottom of the sternum (breastbone). Massage, as taught this week, and the Heart Healing Sound both work to open this point. When this point is closed down you experience impatience, hastiness, cruelty, paranoia and self-pity. When it is open, you feel the positive emotions and qualities of love, joy, happiness, honesty and respect. In time your heart can become the collection point to connect with the source of Universal Love and combine all the positive virtues into compassion.

The final point on the Microcosmic Orbit is the Solar Plexus. This point was previously discussed in Week Eleven, Taoist Self-Massage Rejuvenation. When this point is closed, you can experience panic and worry. When it is open, you feel daring and capable of undertaking risks and challenges.

1. Begin the exercise by focusing on the tip of your nose and then move up to the Third Eye Point.

2. Smile into your eyes and do the Inner Smile.

3. Swallow saliva and follow it with your inner eyes and inner hearing to your Tan Tien. Keep the tip of your tongue raised to the roof of your mouth.

4. Do Bellows Breathing until the Stove at your Tan Tien gets warm.

5. Inhale an Abdominal Breath. Hold for a moment and fix your inner attention on your Tan Tien.

6. Exhale and direct the Energy down to the Sperm/Ovarian Palace, and then down to your Perineum.

7. Inhale a Reverse Breath, and direct the Chi into the sacral hiatus and up your spine, past the Jade Pillow to your Crown Point.

8. Exhale and the Energy flows forward and downward to your Third-Eye Point and then down, through or behind your nose to the roof of your upper palate.

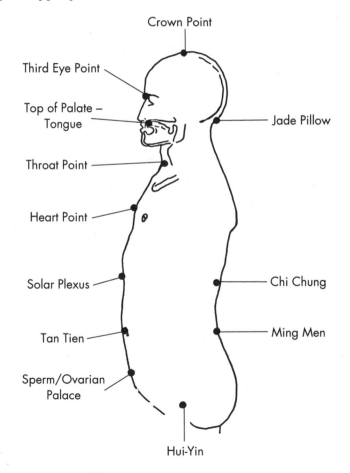

9. The Chi then passes into the raised tip of your tongue, down to your Throat Center and continues down to your Heart Point. Concentrate on the Heart Center for a minute or two.

10. Wash the Channel between the Heart Center and Throat Center six times as you inhale up to the Throat Center and exhale down to the Heart Center.

11. Exhale down from your Heart Center to the Solar Plexus Point. Concentrate here for a minute or two.

12. Wash the Channel between the Solar Plexus Point and the Heart Center 6 times, as you inhale up to the Heart Center and exhale down to the Solar Plexus Point.

13. Exhale down past your Solar Plexus Point to your Tan Tien. Concentrate on your Tan Tien for a minute or so. If you feel the Chi cooling off too much, do some more Bellows Breathing.

14. Wash the Channel between your Tan Tien and your Solar Plexus Point 6 times, inhale up to the Solar Plexus Point and exhale down to the Tan Tien.

15. Exhale down to your Tan Tien and direct the flow of Chi with your Yi Mind, your inner eyesight and your inner hearing down past the Sperm/Ovarian Palace, to your perineum.

16. Inhale a Reverse Breath and guide the Chi through the Governor Channel, all the way up your spine to your Crown Point.

17. Exhale and guide the Chi down past the Third Eye Point and Palate Point and into the tip of your raised tongue and down through all the points on the Functional Channel to your perineum.

18. Continue doing at least 3 more complete Microcosmic Orbits. Inhale a Reverse Breath and direct it from the perineum, up the spine to the Crown Point. Exhale, and direct its flow down and into the Functional Channel to the perineum. When circulating energy in the Orbit, use the navel point as the Tan Tien. When collecting energy, use the interior Tan Tien.

19. When you have finished circulating Chi in the Microcosmic Orbit, collect the Energy at your Tan Tien.

From here on, once you Warm the Stove, you can circulate Chi in the Microcosmic Orbit and coordinate it with Reverse Breathing. Inhale up, exhale down. Some days it will be very powerful. Other days it will feel less powerful. This is normal.

You can also circulate Jing Chi, either aroused, as you learned about this week, or unaroused as you learned about in Seminal/Ovarian Kung Fu in the Microcosmic Orbit. Sexual Energy circulates much more slowly than Chi. Experiment and see if you can feel the difference.

Iron Shirt Packing Process Breathing

YOU HAVE LEARNED MANY BREATHING exercises in this book. One last technique is called Iron Shirt Packing Process Breathing.

Chi **Breath**

Packing Process Breathing increases air pressure inside the body. It is a variation of Reverse Breathing. You take sips of air as you continue to contract your abdomen and use Perineum Power. You force more air into an increasingly smaller space. This increases the Chi Pressure per square inch. The net result is that the Chi is forced into, or literally packed into, the fascia surrounding our organs. This gives us increased strength and wraps our organs in a protective "Iron Shirt." This type of Chi Kung was most important to martial artists who gained the ability to protect the body and organs with a weightless Iron Shirt pressure suit made out of Chi.

This exercise is also important in the rooting process. The more you can root into Mother Earth the more balanced your Energy will be, which in turn increases your own healing energy.

The position we will use is essentially the same position you learned in Yi Chin Ching: The Muscle-Tendon Change Classic, except your arms are held at shoulder height in front of you as if you were embracing a large tree. Master Tseng has told me that there are over 300 different forms of Chi Kung in China today. Of these, more than ninety percent use this form. I first learned it from Master Mantak Chia as part of Iron Shirt Chi Kung. You will learn a simplified version of the first position known as Embracing the Tree.

This exercise also introduces a new dimension in Perineum Power. For the first time we pull up on the left and right sides of the anus. This allows us to send Energy up the sides of our body. We will send it to our left and right kidneys.

1. Stand with feet shoulder width apart. You claw the ground with the toes of your feet. Activate the Sacral and Cranial Pumps and round your shoulders as your arms are held in front of you and you Embrace the Tree.

2. Your fingertips face each other and your thumbs are held up and pushed slightly forward, away from your body as your pinkies are pushed slightly toward your body. This increases the tension in the tendons of your hands and forearms. Your palms are in front of your face.

3. Begin with a few Abdominal Breaths.

4. Exhale and contract your lower abdomen.

5. Inhale a small sip of air, maybe 10 percent of your normal capacity. Keep your lower abdomen flat.

6. Take a second sip of air. Push down on your diaphragm, use Perineum Power and pull up on your sexual organs and anus and pull in the lower abdomen. This compresses the abdominal organs in three directions: from above, from below, and from the front. Keep your chest relaxed.

7. Inhale another 10 percent sip of air. Contract the left side of your anus. Direct Chi to rise up the left side of your body to your left kidney. Wrap the left kidney, and the adrenal gland that sits on top of it, with Chi and pack the Chi into the left kidney as you pull in the left side of your stomach.

8. Inhale another 10 percent sip of air. Contract the right side of your anus. Direct Chi to rise up the right side of your body to your right kidney. Wrap the right kidney, and the adrenal gland that sits on top of it, with Chi and pack the Chi into the right kidney as you pull in the right side of your stomach.

9. Pack and wrap the Energy around both kidneys. Pull in both sides of the stomach. Hold this position as long as you can, a few seconds at least.

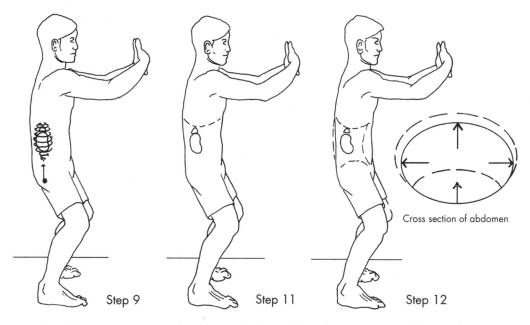

Cross section of abdomen

Step 9   Step 11   Step 12

10. When you run out of breath, inhale another 10 percent sip of air and contract the perineum and anus even more tightly. Feel the pressure expand into the Sperm/Ovarian Palace area.

11. Inhale another 10 percent sip of air. Contract the pelvic area and lower part of the diaphragm and hold this position as long as you can. Feel the pressure build in the perineum area.

12. Exhale a small amount of air, then bend slightly forward at the waist and inhale another 10 percent sip of air. Direct your attention back to your kidneys and push outward in the kidney area. Feel them actually expand on both sides and backward.

13. Inhale the last 10 percent sip of air to the kidney area of your back. Hold as long as possible.

14. Exhale and stand up straight. Use Bellows Breathing to normalize your breath.

15. In the beginning, don't do more than 3 times a day.

16. Optional: To finish the exercise you can send the energy you have created in this exercise into the Microcosmic Orbit by raising the tip of your tongue to the roof of your mouth. Do a few Orbits then collect the Energy at your navel.

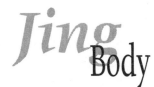

Taoist Self-Massage Rejuvenation

YOU'VE LEARNED SO MUCH in this book. I've saved this last chapter for some of my Taoist Self-Massage Rejuvenation personal favorites.

Inner Eardrum Blowing Exercise

The first one helps to clear your inner ears when they feel stuffy or under pressure. I often use it when I'm listening to music and the music sounds fuzzy. One or two blasts of this exercise and my hearing is usually crystal clear.

This exercise makes use of swallowing the breath as you learned in Week Twelve, Compression Breathing.

1. Inhale deeply, filling the lower abdomen, middle lungs, upper lungs, and into your throat.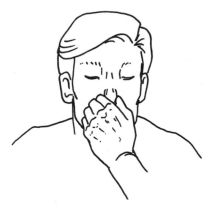

2. Swallow the breath with a gulping sound.

3. Pinch your nostrils closed with the thumb and index finger of either hand.

4. Blow (exhale) gently into your closed-off nostrils. The pressure will slowly build up and move into both ear canals. Often you will hear your ear drums popping.

5. Swallow the breath again with a gulping sound.

6. Release your fingers from your nose and exhale slowly through your nose. Do a total of 2 or 3 times.

Don't blow into your nostrils too hard. This could injure your inner ear. Blow gently, but firmly. This also exercises your inner ear and helps to maintain and establish your equilibrium.

Swinging the Arms

This is a simple and basic exercise that really helps to loosen up the muscles and tendons of the arms and shoulders and gets your Chi flowing.

1. Start with your arms hanging at your sides.

2. Swing your left arm forward, up and around like a windmill, 360 degrees. Do this at least 6 times.

3. Reverse and swing your left arm backwards, up and around 360 degrees. Do this at least 6 times.

4. Repeat with your right arm in both directions.

Just make sure you have sufficient room before you start swinging. Keep your arms relaxed as you swing them. Don't tense them up.

Shaking Out the Body

This is an exercise that should be done at the conclusion of every Chi Kung exercise session. Just stand in one spot and bounce up and down on your feet and toes as you shake out your hands and arms. Move around as much as you want. You can bend your knees as you bounce. Just remember to shake.

Flick out your hands and fingers. Twist to the left and to the right as you bounce up and down. Do it for 30 seconds or a minute. It will help to keep you flexible and loose.

Tao In: Part Five

Tao In Breathing

Rather than learn any more Tao In forms, instead, this final week, you will learn the important practice of Tao In Breathing.

The Taoists believed that seventy percent of the toxins in the body are eliminated through the breath when we exhale. Sometimes it is difficult for certain parts of the body to receive sufficient oxygen, blood and Chi to help remove all the toxins in the cells.

The Taoists developed techniques to breathe directly into different parts of the body. This is another longtime oral secret practice that works to relax and heal the body, and remove toxins.

Tao In Breathing relies on your ability to direct your concentration to specific parts of your body. By this final stage of the 100 Days of Practice this should pose no difficulty for you. You have learned to guide Chi with your Yi Mind, your inner eyesight, inner hearing, breath, and through movement. If you remember back to Week Five, you also learned to direct Chi with the palms of your hands. The Tiger and Dragon Cavities in the middle of your palms are the strongest points for moving or guiding Chi. When the two palms are placed over each other with the Dragon Cavity of the right palm placed over the back of the left palm, directly in line with the Tiger Cavity of the left hand (if you are a man or the Tiger Cavity over the Dragon Cavity of the right hand if you are a woman), they reinforce each other and act like lenses to direct the flow of Chi. You will make use of this ability in Tao In Breathing.

When you do Tao In Breathing, it is important to relax. Once your body is totally relaxed, you will then direct Chi to different locations in your body and place your palms, with the Dragon and Tiger Cavities aligned, over the area. If you are sufficiently relaxed and quiet inside, it feels as if you are breathing right into the part of the body you are directing the Energy to. It also feels as though you are inhaling and exhaling right through the skin. You feel a smiling, loving and healing Energy pass directly into you.

Once you learn the basic exercise, I'll give you some more details about the healing aspect of Tao In Breathing.

1. Lie flat on your back on a firm surface.

2. Do deep, slow, Abdominal Breathing. To help you slow down you can use the technique you learned in Week One. Inhale and mentally tell yourself "calm" and exhale and mentally say "relaxed." Do this for a few minutes until you are calm and relaxed.

3. *Men:* Place your left palm over your navel and place your right palm on top of the left, with the Dragon and Tiger Cavities aligned. *Women:* Place your right palm over your navel and place your left palm on top of the right, with the Tiger and Dragon Cavities aligned. For the remainder of this exercise, no matter where you move them, keep the palms aligned in this manner.

4. Inhale and feel or imagine that Chi and air are being drawn from above (Heavenly Energy) and is passing right into your navel. The Energy passing into you is smiling, loving, healing Chi.

5. Exhale and you breathe out of your navel. As you do this breathing, your skin expands and contracts like rubber. Do this breathing at the navel for a minute or more.

6. Move your palms down to your Sperm/Ovarian Palace and repeat as above.

7. Cover your sexual organs with your palms and breathe into your sexual organs as above.

8. Move your palms up to your diaphragm/solar plexus area and repeat here.

9. Next cover the lower part of your chest and breathe through the skin.

10. Move to the upper part of your chest and repeat.

11. Place your palms over your throat and imagine or feel the Chi pass right through your palms all the way to the back of your neck.

12. Place your palms over your Third Eye Point, and imagine or feel the Chi pass all the way through your head to the Jade Pillow at the base of the skull.

13. The final position is your Crown Point. Cover it with both palms aligned as before and breathe into your Crown Point.

Do the exercise slowly and you will actually begin to feel as if you can breathe right through your skin. It is helpful to use inner hearing and direct it to the spot and listen to yourself breathing. The quieter your breathing, the better it works. Absolutely silent breathing is best. Tao In Breathing can be used to direct Chi to any part of your body. Just cover any spot you wish to affect or heal with your aligned palms and breathe into that spot. If there are certain spots that you can only reach with one palm (for instance, the under-arm area), do so, but try to send Chi to the spot with your other palm even though it is not in direct contact.

It might take you some time and practice before you feel the Chi pass through your skin. Remember, the quieter you can make your breathing, the easier this practice becomes. When your breathing becomes totally silent, this exercise will become easy to do.

Learning to breathe directly into our body helps that area to regain tone and resiliency. Use your Yi Mind to direct the Energy. When you direct Chi to a part of the body, this also causes the blood flow to increase to that same point. This increased blood circulation might partially explain the healing aspects of Tao In Breathing. Experiment with it. With the proper open-minded attitude of the Taoist, breathing through the skin has a delightful, childlike quality to it.

Sexual Kung Fu: Dual Cultivation

Dual Cultivation is a vast field of knowledge and practice. The basic premise of all these practices is balancing the Yin and Yang Energies.

The old-time Taoist practices are in large part inappropriate for modern times. They often involved one man having intercourse with numerous women in a single evening. As soon as the male felt himself getting sufficiently aroused, he would change partners. Throughout the evening he would refrain from ejaculating. After hours of ecstasy, the evening would fade into sleepy oblivion or an energized sunrise.

Although the above would appear to be every male's fantasy and every feminist's nightmare, a little bit of theory will help to understand what was happening from an Energy point of view. I have no opinion as to the propriety of these practices. They occurred in a different time, in a different culture, with different values and mindset than exist today. For Dual Cultivation to work, the male must absorb the female Energy and the female must absorb the male Energy. Here are the olden secrets about this Energy.

Feminine Sexual Energy is not lost through orgasm. It actually increases when aroused. This Feminine Sexual Energy also increases geometrically with each additional female added to the experience, as long as there is a male present. Thus, two women will create a field of charged Sexual Energy that is four times as powerful as one woman. Three women will create a field of Sexual Energy that is eight times as powerful as a solo woman. And so on. The preferred number among the Taoists seemed to be three or five women, although some ancient sources say ten. The women would be engaged in lovemaking between themselves and the male.

Into this sexually charged field of energy, we find a single male Taoist, not two or three. There are two basic reasons for this. For one, this sexual encounter is entered into for health and longevity purposes and not to satisfy carnal desires. Secondly, male Sexual Energy is limited. Two or more males will tend to cancel out each other's Sexual Energy. Evidence of this is found in the fact that if you mix sperm cells of different males together, the different sperm cells will actually fight with each other. A Yang sexual field of such initial intensity will be created that will generally quickly burn itself out in male orgasm and the total loss of any of the beneficial effects gained.

A single male could take advantage of the intense sexual field created with the multiple female partners, if he was able to control his orgasm and ejaculation. His Yang Jing Chi would continue to expand in intensity as long as he didn't ejaculate. The women, in turn, could absorb the highly aroused male Sexual Energy and also benefit from the balancing and healing Energy field that had been created by the interaction of the man and the women and the women with the women. The Yin and Yang Energies were balanced. Nobody was a loser. Everyone came out of these sessions a winner. This all took place in a culture that was unaware of the concept of Original Sin or sexual guilt.

In old times one Taoist male and many female partners was not considered an orgy, it was considered to be medicine. The Bedroom Arts were part of traditional Chinese medicine until they were suppressed by a prudish, conservative dynasty a thousand years ago. These Bedroom Arts developed very definite rules and regulations. There were numerous sexual positions used to cure different ailments and illnesses. Imagine having sex prescribed by your Taoist physician to regain and maintain your health. I just love the Taoist mentality! For all intents and purposes, opportunities for one male and multiple female partners, although not impossible, are just not a realistic lifestyle in our modern world.

To the modern Taoist, the mindset is somewhat different from the ancient sage's. Each woman has an inexhaustible fountain of Sexual Energy available to her. If this Energy is properly handled, then sexuality can be used to strengthen, heal and form an incredibly uniting bond between the woman and a man. It is not necessary for the man to require multiple female partners. Instead, the basic modern rule is for the woman to have multiple orgasms while the man does not ejaculate, although he may have an orgasm and block the Million Dollar Point, conserving all or most of his semen. Use of the Big Draw and the Orgasmic Upward Draw makes Dual Cultivation feasible, and I've already taught you how to do that by yourself. You just have to learn how to do it with a partner.

It is impossible for me to describe all the implications and possibilities of Dual Cultivation in one week's lesson. What I would like to do is give you enough information so that you and your partner can begin.

Setting the Mood

Dual Cultivation is predicated upon lovemaking sessions lasting an hour, two hours or more. Setting the proper mood is helpful to get things started.

Nothing elaborate is really required. If the room you are using is a mess, cleaning it up beforehand creates a setting more conducive to controlled lovemaking.

A burning candle or dim lights should also be used if the session is at night. You should be able to see your partner. Total darkness is not conducive to lengthy Taoist sex.

Soft music, New Age music or light jazz is often helpful, depending on your and your partner's taste. Hard rock or other forms of loud, pulsing music are too emotionally and physically arousing and should be avoided.

A glass of wine will help you relax, warm up inside and get in the mood. I said a glass of wine—well, maybe two. Any more will interfere with your ability to concentrate and perform.

Mantak Chia recommends erotic movies if this is not offensive to your part-ner. The sights and sounds of men and women having sex is very stimulating to some people, and a turn-off to others. If the movies get the male too aroused so that he cannot control his orgasm, they should be avoided.

If you are aware of personal things to do to set the proper mood for you and your partner, then by all means do them. Each of us is different, with different tastes and preferences. Cater to them.

Foreplay

Foreplay plays a major role in Taoist sex. Beginning with a mental attitude of slow, relaxed sex, foreplay can go on for a long period of time before you actu-ally engage in intercourse, sometimes for an hour or two, or more.

It is most important to have the male and the female fully aroused. Old Taoist texts give lists of the various stages of sexual excitement for men and women. The bottom line though is that both partners must be fully aroused. If only the man is aroused and hard and the female is still dry, then the time has not arrived yet for intercourse. If the woman is wet and wild but the man is still limp, you're also not ready. The Taoists call this "dead fish meeting the water."

Foreplay is a difficult subject to write about because different things turn on different people. Of course touching, tender caresses and kissing are always a good way to start.

The Taoists believed that saliva had healing and balancing qualities. Swallow-ing your partner's saliva as you kiss is one of the most basic means of Yin-Yang Energy exchange that can take place between men and women. Sucking on your partner's tongue was especially recommended for a man to perform on a woman, both for its erotic feel (don't suck too hard) and because this stimulated the flow of saliva from underneath her tongue. The Taoists referred to the female tongue as the Red Lotus Peak and its medicine (saliva) was called Jade Liquid.

Massaging, caressing, kneading, licking and sucking on the woman's breast is another cornerstone of foreplay. A woman's nipple is often overly sensitive before the woman herself is fully aroused. So avoid squeezing or pinching her nipples until she is obviously aroused and her nipples are erect. The Taoists believed that a medicine or elixir issued forth from the woman's nipples or Twin Lotus Chestnuts. This medicine was referred to as White Snow. When a man sucks on the woman's nipple and swallows the White Snow, it strength-ens his spleen and his Third Treasure, Shen. Although Taoist texts refer to its color as white and to its taste as sweet and delicate, this is poetic license, it cannot really be seen by the outer eyes. It was definitely not mother's milk because the same text says that a woman who has never had a baby has the most potent Chestnuts. I'm not sure if that's still true today. Sucking on a woman's nipples will also open her Chi meridians, relax her mind and body and stimulate the flow of sexual fluids in her vagina.

Tongue Kung Fu, which I introduced to you in Week Four, works very nicely on the breasts and nipples. But you should all know that by now.

Men's nipples are generally overlooked in Western sexual literature. They are not a well-established part of our sexual culture. However, once the male is highly aroused, his nipples can also be erotically stimulating. In the Taoist literature, a woman sucking on a man's nipple was a sure sign of extreme feminine arousal.

In Taoist lore, women have Three Peaks of Great Medicine: the tongue, the nipples and the vagina. The Chinese referred to this last Peak as the Jade Fountain, Cave of the White Tiger or the Mysterious Gate, to name but a few. Its medicine was called Moon Flower. This is what Tongue Kung Fu was created for. Any man with due diligence can become a master of this domain. Personal hygiene is really important here. The intake of Moon Flower strengthens a man's Yang Energy and also nourishes his Third Treasure, Spirit, which is the higher form of Shen.

Of course, not to be forgotten, is the practice of Playing the Flute. In the literature of Sexual Alchemy it is said that Playing the Flute opens the pathway up the spine, allowing Jing Chi to be converted into Chi and rise up the spine to the Crown Point (Pai Hui) where it is converted into Shen, Spiritual Energy. Thus the woman performing oral sex on her male partner was an important part of Dual Cultivation, from an Energy point of view.

Playing the Flute also stimulates the woman and helps to open her Mysterious Gate (gets her aroused and her sexual fluids flowing). The original Taoist literature gives little in the way of technique for fellatio. Of course use Tongue Kung Fu but this is not enough. I will leave you to your own devices here with but three rules: 1. Do it; 2. Don't bite; and 3. Don't excite your partner until he reaches the point of no return and ejaculates (if you do, I implore you to keep trying until you get it right).

Using your hand and fingers to explore and masturbate your partner's genitals is a standard part of foreplay. Some couples are also excited by watching their partner masturbate.

The aim of foreplay is to get both participants hot, really turned on. This is especially true of the woman. If she can be brought to orgasm once or twice before intercourse begins, so much the better. But the man, though aroused, must keep a cool head and avoid ejaculation. If he starts to lose it, be sure he uses the Three Finger Method and block the Million Dollar Point. This isn't usually 100 percent effective, but it should conserve forty to eighty percent of the Jing Chi that would otherwise be lost. In the old practices the Sexual Energy field created by one man and multiple women was easy to ignite. Creating this type of highly charged Sexual Energy field between one man and one woman can be achieved if you both work at it. What could be more fun than that?

Intercourse

We have three goals here: 1. To have long, slow, sensuous sex; 2. To draw Sexual Energy up to the head using the Big Draw or the Orgasmic Upward Draw; and 3. To exchange Energy with our partner.

To achieve lengthy sex, the Taoist teachings recommend that the woman be the more active partner and the man the more passive. An often recommended position was the woman on top. The male was encouraged to keep his mind calm, so as not to lose control and ejaculate. Techniques for long and short thrusts of the penis into the vagina were often used. The most popular was the so-called Nine to One Method, which allowed for nine shallow thrusts followed by one deep thrust. It's hard to ejaculate when you're counting. It is also tremendously stimulating to the woman. Try starting with three to one, three shallow and one deep and see what happens. You might like it.

When the man is close to orgasm, he must stop thrusting and withdraw his penis so that only the head is inside the vagina. This will place it in close contact to the woman's so-called G-spot. Squeeze the urogenital diaphragm at the base of the penis as tight as you can and do the Big Draw. Tighten your buttocks, clench your teeth, push your tongue to the roof of your mouth, clench both fists and press them down toward your feet. Hold your breath, use your Sacral and Cranial Pumps and contract the entire perineum area nine times as you look up toward your Crown Point and draw the Sexual Energy up the spine, through the neck and into your head. When your penis begins to soften, start slowly thrusting again.

The female partner must be aware of what the male is doing and refrain from trying to push the male over the orgasmic brink when he is trying to apply the Big Draw. Once the male has completed his first round of Big Draw his body fills with hot Yang Energy. Now it is time for the woman to use the Orgasmic Upward Draw. There will be an exchange of male Jing Chi into the woman as she stops moving and allows the male's penis to withdraw so that just the head is gripped tightly by the vaginal muscles, in contact with her G-spot. Do the

Orgasmic Upward Draw. Tighten the lips of the vagina. Tighten your buttocks, clench your teeth, push your tongue to the roof of your mouth, clench both fists and press them down toward your feet. Hold your breath, use your Sacral and Cranial Pumps and contract the entire perineum area nine times, look up toward your Crown Point and draw the Sexual Energy up the spine, through the neck and into your head.

When you have completed the first round of Big Draw and Orgasmic Upward Draw, you are ready for the second round. The Taoists claimed that the ability to do ten rounds without the male ejaculating led to immortality. Wouldn't you like to try it and find out?

Partners share and exchange Energy when they do the Big Draw and Orgasmic Upward Draw. Energy can also be passed through the hands and led up your partner's spine as you embrace.

If you can synchronize your breathing with your partner, you can exchange balancing Sexual Energy. Either partner can start. One partner, let's say the male, exhales and directs Sexual Energy in his breath to the female partner who inhales this Sexual Energy and then she in turn exhales as the male inhales. Go on for as long as you like. You can also use this method during foreplay.

Joining your Microcosmic Orbit with your partner's is the final technique we will discuss. There are many ways to do this. I will describe the most common and easiest method.

The Figure-Eight Method

1. Engage in sexual intercourse.

2. Place your mouths together and kiss. The Energy passes through your tongue, which acts like a switch.

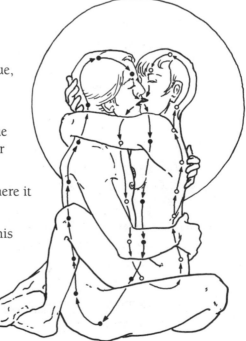

Men:

3. The Energy goes from the man's tongue into the woman's mouth and down her throat into the Functional Channel.

4. The Energy descends to her vagina where it passes into the male's penis.

5. The male draws the Energy back up his spine, to his Crown, Third Eye and tongue and then passes the Energy back to the female through his tongue, to start another round of the Microcosmic Orbit.

Women:

3. The Energy goes from the woman's tongue into the man's mouth and down his throat in the Functional Channel.

4. The Energy descends to his penis where it passes into the female's vagina.

5. The female draws the Energy back up her spine, to her Crown, Third Eye and tongue and then passes the Energy back to the male through her tongue to start another round of the Microcosmic Orbit.

Opening the Golden Flower

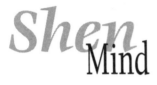

WE'VE FINALLY ARRIVED AT THE last practice of these 100 Days of Practice. This one is something special. It has a whole different flavor than anything else I've given you in this book. It has the true quality of the oral tradition and is in harmony with the Tao. It can be done sitting or standing in the Embracing the Tree stance.

1. Focus on the tip of your nose. Then bring your concentration up to the Third Eye.

2. Visualize a smiling Moon, smiling into your eyes. Smile into the inner and outer corners, the pupils, irises, whites and upper and lower lids. Raise the corners of your lips and relax your face and eyes.

3. Smile into your heart, your lungs, your liver, your kidneys and your spleen.

4. Make saliva in your mouth. Smile into the saliva. Swallow the saliva. Guide the smiling Energy down through your digestive system.

5. Smile into the left side of your brain, then the right side of your brain. Smile down the center of your brain to the base of your skull. Smile down your spine, vertebra by vertebra.

6. Return your awareness to the Third Eye. Turn your inner eyesight upward and backward toward the Crown Point.

7. Visualize a full Moon over your head. See it perfectly round and white or silvery white. Let it hang there for a minute or two as you slowly do Abdominal Breathing.

8. The Moon starts to slowly descend. It surrounds your head as it inches downward.

9. The Moon descends and encircles your entire neck area. It continues down surrounding your chest.

10. As you look inward and downward with your inner eyes, you see the Moon reach the level of your solar plexus. Just below your solar plexus you can see still waters, like the surface of a motionless lake.

11. You see the moonlight reflecting off the water's surface. Slowly the Moon sinks down through the surface of the water.

12. You look down and see the Moon under the still surface of the water.

13. Begin doing Bellows Breathing. As you continue doing this, your Tan Tien grows hotter. You look down and realize that you were looking at a reflection. There, where the Moon was, you now see the Sun. See it expand, growing brighter and brighter.

14. After experiencing the Sun in your Tan Tien for a minute or two, see the Sun start to contract. It continues to contract and condense until it is just a tiny dot or pearl of Sunlight.

15. Allow the tiny glowing pearl of Sunlight to descend to your perineum.

16. Inhale a Reverse Breath and the tiny dot of glowing Sunlight shoots up your Governor Channel to your Crown.

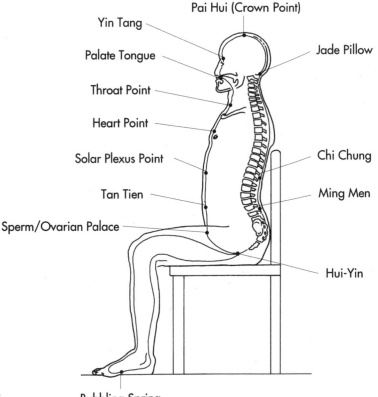

17. Exhale and the Sunlight pearl descends down your Functional Channel. In this same manner, circulate the tiny pearl of Sunlight in your Microcosmic Orbit.

18. After a few circulations, inhale and bring the pearl to your Crown Point, then exhale and the tiny Sunlight pearl descends down the Functional Channel to your perineum where it splits in two and descends down the front of your legs, over the top of your feet and circles over the toes to the Bubbling Spring, behind the ball of your foot.

19. Inhale a Reverse Breath and the Chi rises from your heels up the back of your legs to your perineum where it joins together and shoots up the Governor Channel to your Crown Point.

20. Do a few complete circulations including going down and up your legs. This is called the Macrocosmic Orbit.

21. Return the tiny glowing pearl of Sunlight to your Tan Tien. Do some deep, slow Abdominal Breaths and see the tiny pearl begin to grow. It turns into a Golden Flower that opens and blossoms in your Tan Tien and floats on the still waters like a lotus.

22. Relax and breathe deeply. After a minute or two the Golden Flower fades away.

23. Collect the energy at your navel. Rub your hands together and massage your face. Rub your hands together again and cover your eyes. Absorb the Chi into your eyes.

The Macrocosmic Orbit connects the legs to the Microcosmic Orbit. The Moon is Yin Energy. The Sun is Yang Energy. In this Meditation we combined the Sun and the Moon and created a tiny seed pearl that grows and blossoms into the Golden Flower. The Golden Flower sprouts and blossoms in the "Elixir Field" or Tan Tien. Its appearance represents a whole new level of your body being able to heal and protect itself, as well as a definite and profound increase in your Third Treasure—in this case, Spiritual Energy, as well as Mental Energy. What this ultimately means to us is different for each person. But it is always a positive sign. And thus our 100 Days of Practice draw to a close.

One final note on the Microcosmic Orbit. Sometimes it is hard to move. If this happens, reverse the direction of the flow and bring it up the Functional Channel, over the head and down the Governor Channel. It's not a bad idea to do this a few times every week. This helps to balance your Yin and Yang Energies and keeps your Chi from stagnating from only traveling in one direction.

It is important to grow comfortable with sensing and directing the flow of Energy in your body. Experiment, be creative and have fun. Most important, practice every day and return to this book as you would to an old dear friend. In time your compassionate heart may come to encompass the whole world as you nurture your greatest possession.

道

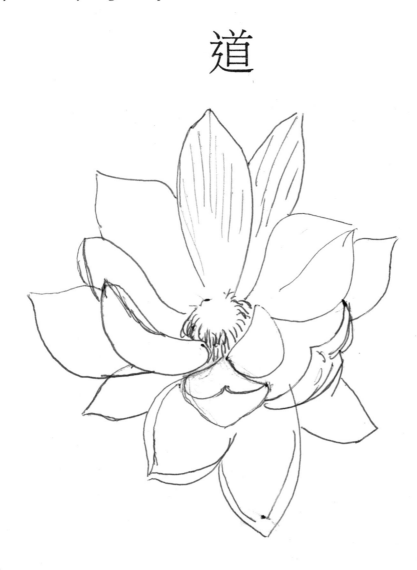

conclusion

So, NOW YOU'VE FINISHED THE 100 Days of Practice. I hope you found it worthwhile. You've learned new ideas and had experiences that few Westerners before you have ever encountered.

If you've done the exercises diligently, you must realize that your adventure with the Tao is just beginning. There is really enough material in this book to keep you busy for the rest of your life. You have built a basic foundation of Taoist health, longevity, rejuvenation and sexual practices. I invite you to return to this book many times and review what you have learned. You didn't come this far just to stop because there are no more pages to read. I assure you that there will always be something here that you have forgotten or will now seem more important as you continue in your practice. When you go back, apply what you learned in the later weeks of practice and the earlier exercises will often take on a whole new meaning for you. Have fun with the Energy.

You have built a foundation in the practice of Taoist Yoga. This self-cultivation allows us to, little by little, slag off the darkness and debris that has attached itself to us as we grew up, and to uncover our true Original Nature. Once the foundation is established, the path develops.

Each of us is born with an Original Nature untainted and uncorrupted as yet by contact with the world and the ideas we will come to learn from our parents, friends, teachers, relatives and all the other people who will influence us, either consciously or unconsciously. The light of the Golden Flower will gradually wear away, melt and dissolve all these accumulations to your Original Nature. It was said by the ancient Taoists that once a person was born, he or she moves away from his Original Nature. You now have the means to begin to reverse this process and restore your Original Nature, which includes cultivation of your true natural talents and abilities.

To progress in Taoist Yoga and aid in the restoration of your Original Nature, it is necessary to cultivate your own moral character. You must strive to become what the I Ching calls the Superior Man or Woman. You must seek to do good for its own sake, not for any reward. Strive to be the best person you can be. When in doubt, ask Heaven what is right. The positive emotions and virtues of the organs and elements that you learned earlier in this book must come to replace any negative emotions that rule you. This will happen gradually. Slow, steady progress leads eventually to great rewards.

When you lose contact with your Original Nature, you also lose your connection to the Universe and thus sever yourself from the source of life. In this book I have sought to reconnect you to the silent source of life called the Tao. Remember: Life is your greatest possession.

May the Chi be with you.

道

Tranquility of mind lets me live long,
Smiling keeps me always young.
I am air,
I am light,
And I am Water.
With the breeze I drift,
Far and wide.

—Chen Yan-feng

from *Prenatal Energy Mobilising Qigong—China Taoist Ancient Qigong* (sic), Guangdong Science and Technology Press, Guangzhou, China, 1992.

glossary

Abdominal Breath: A type of breath in which the diaphragm is pushed down and the lower abdomen is expanded upon inhalation. The diaphragm is relaxed and lower abdomen is contracted upon exhalation.

Aura: Electromagnetic energy field surrounding the body.

Backward Flowing Method: Taoist techniques for reversing the normal flow of various bodily functions, such as directing the eyesight inward or having sexual energy flow upward rather than out of the body.

Baduanjin (the Eight Pieces of Brocade): A set of eight simple Chi Kung exercises originally developed to keep soldiers in the field fit and limber.

Bellows Breathing: Rapid Abdominal Breathing used to raise heat in the Lower Tan Tien (Warming the Stove). Also called *Quick Fire*.

Big Draw: A sexual exercise for men designed to raise aroused sexual energy to the brain.

Breatharians: Legendary Tao Masters who achieved immortality and sustained their bodies on breath alone.

Bubbling Spring (Yong Quan): An energy point on the bottom of the foot, at the indentation at the rear of the ball of the foot. Used to draw Energy (Chi) up the legs (Sole Breathing) or down into the ground.

Chi: The First Treasure of Taoist Yoga. Breath. Air. Energy. Often referred to as Life Force Energy, the energy of life itself. A word with many subtle and different meanings in Chinese.

Chi Chung: A point on the Governor Channel located on the spine opposite the solar plexus (T-11).

Chi Kung: Originally breathing exercises. Now a generic name for exercises combining movement, breathing and mentally directing Energy (Chi).

257

Cranial Pump: A "pump" located at the point where the back of the skull and top of the neck meet. It is used to pump Energy (Chi) or Essence (Jing) up the Governor Channel and into the head. It is activated by pulling in the chin and straightening the back of the neck.

Crystal Palace: The major energy center in the brain, consisting of the area encompassing the pituitary, pineal, thalamus and hypothalamus glands. It is activated through the various processes of Taoist Yoga. It is where enlightenment takes place. Also called the *Upper Tan Tien* or *Heavenly Heart.*

Dragon Cavity: An energy center in the palm of the right hand, located by bending the middle finger into the palm. Used to absorb or send out Chi (Energy).

Dual Cultivation: Taoist sexual practices involving a male and female participant.

Earth: One of the Five Elements (Five Forces). It is a neutral element with a stabilizing force. It is associated with the spleen and pancreas and its color is yellow or golden yellow.

Earth Chi: The Energy that exists inside our planet.

Emotional Mind: See *Hsin.*

Energy: See *Chi.*

Energy Channels (Energy Meridians): Often referred to as acupuncture channels. The pathways in the body that Chi circulates through.

Essence: See *Jing.*

Fire: One of the Five Elements (Five Forces). It is hot active energy associated with the heart and the color red.

First Treasure: Breath (Chi). One of the three basic components of Taoist Yoga.

Five Elements (Five Forces): The five basic forms of energy of which the physical universe is composed. They are Fire, Water, Wood, Metal and Earth.

Functional Channel (Ren Mai): One of the body's two main Energy Channels. It is located at the front of the body running from the tip of the tongue to the perineum.

Golden Flower (Secret of the): Activated Energy in the Upper Tan Tien in the brain and Lower Tan Tien (Medicine Field) located behind and below the navel. It is associated with the body's ability to maintain good health and long life as well as higher consciousness. The activation of the Golden Flower is a prime goal of Taoist Yoga.

Governor Channel (Du Mai): One of the body's two main Energy Channels. It is located on the back of the body as well as in the skull. It runs from the perineum up the spine and over the skull to the upper palate behind the teeth.

Heavenly Chi: Energy that exists above the earth including the energy of the sun, moon, planets and stars as well as cosmic rays, meteors, comets and any other energy that falls to earth from above.

Heavenly Heart: The higher mind (Yi Mind). Associated with the intellect, will and higher consciousness. It is located in the brain and is also called the *Upper Tan Tien* or *Crystal Palace*.

Heavenly Pool: The soft palate located at the top rear of the inner mouth. It is directly below the pituitary gland.

Hegu: A point on the hand between the thumb and index finger. It is often sore and responds well to massage.

Hsin (Emotional Mind): That aspect of the mind that is ruled by the emotions. It is associated with the human heart rather than the brain.

Human Chi: Energy that exists on the surface of the earth as opposed to above (Heavenly Chi) or below (Earth Chi).

I Ching (The Book of Changes): Oldest existing Chinese text, it is both a book of wisdom and divination. Its teachings set out the way of life for the Superior Man or Woman.

Immortal: A Tao Master who has achieved the ability to have his consciousness (Spirit-Shen) leave his body at will and exist independent of his body. Also refers to a Taoist who has achieved extreme old age.

Inner Smile: Taoist technique for activating the eyes and internal organs using smiling energy.

Internal Alchemy: Taoist processes for altering the internal energies within the body. These are more advanced practices that are not covered in this book.

Iron Shirt Packing Process Breathing: A breathing exercise. A form of Reverse Breathing in which Chi is packed into the internal organs so as to wrap them in an internal "iron shirt."

Jade Pillow: A point on the Governor Channel at the base of the skull.

Jing (Essence): The Second Treasure of Taoist Yoga. Refers to the body and bodily fluids including sexual organs and fluids.

Jing Chi: Sexual Energy.

Life Force Energy: See *Chi*.

Lower Tan Tien: Principal Energy field in the body. Literally lower "elixir" or "medicine" field. Located approximately two finger widths below the navel and halfway to two-thirds of the way between the navel and the spine.

Macrocosmic Orbit: Combines circulating Chi in the Microcosmic Orbit (Governor and Functional Channels) with circulation up and down the legs.

Metal: One of the Five Elements (Five Forces). It is cool, dry energy associated with the lungs. Its color is metallic white.

Microcosmic Orbit: The basic energy circuit of the body. It is formed by circulating Chi through the body's two main Energy Channels—the Governor and Functional Channel. The circuit is completed by raising the tip of the tongue to the upper palate behind the teeth.

Million Dollar Point: A point in the perineum that is pressed with the fingers just before or during male orgasm, to prevent or lessen the ejaculation of sperm.

Ming Men: A point on the Governor Channel opposite the navel.

Muscle Tendon Change Classic: See *Yi Chin Ching*.

Nectar (Heavenly Nectar): Sweet tasting flow of energy that drips onto the raised tongue from the brain. A result of the brain filling with raised Sexual Energy (Jing Chi).

Nei Dan: Internal exercises.

Nei Kung: Internal Power. Building strength from the inside out, rather than the outside in, as in traditional Western exercises.

Ocean of Chi: See *Sea of Chi*.

Orgasmic Upward Draw: Sexual exercise for women to draw aroused sexual energy to the brain.

Original Chi (Yuan Chi): The energy that provides the spark of life. It will sustain us from the time of conception and slowly weaken until the moment of death. Restoring Original Chi is the prime goal of Taoist Yoga. Also called *Vital Energy (Force)*.

Original Jing (Yuan Jing): The Original Essence received from the union of our parents' egg and sperm. It is converted into Original Chi to provide the energy of life.

Original Nature: Who and what we really are, including natural talents and abilities, when stripped of the corrupting influence of contact with the world and the thoughts and ideas we learn from our parents, friends, teachers and all other people who influence us, either consciously or unconsciously.

Ovarian Breathing: A sexual practice for women to raise unaroused Sexual Energy (Jing Chi) to the head.

Ovarian Compression: A female breathing and sexual practice for flooding the sexual organs with Chi.

Ovarian Kung Fu: Taoist sexual practices for women.

Ovarian Palace: A point on the woman's Functional Channel just above the vagina.

Perenium Power: Strengthening the perineum, the point between the sexual organs and the anus, to increase the body's strength and its ability to conserve and direct Energy (Chi) within the body.

Playing the Flute: Fellatio. Oral sex performed on the male sexual organ.

Power Lock Exercise: Generic name for the male Big Draw and female Orgasmic Upward Draw.

Quick Fire: See *Bellows Breathing*.

Reverse Breathing: Breathing technique in which the diaphragm is pushed down and the lower abdomen is contracted upon inhalation. Both are relaxed upon exhalation.

Sacral Pump: Using the sacrum at the bottom of the spine to pump Jing or Chi up the spine.

Scapula Power: Using the shoulder blades to move the arms rather then the muscles of the arms.

Scrotal Compression: A male breathing and sexual practice for flooding the sexual organs with Energy (Chi).

Sea of Chi: The body's main reservoir of Chi. It is located behind the navel in the lower abdomen and includes the Lower Tan Tien. Also called *Ocean of Chi.*

Second Treasure: The body essence (Jing). The second of the three basic components of Taoist Yoga.

Self-Massage Rejuvenation: Simple exercises and self-massage techniques to revitalize specific parts of the body.

Seminal Kung Fu: Taoist sexual practices for men.

Sexual Kung Fu: Taoist sexual practices.

Sick Winds: Air and gases that are trapped in the body, which cause various ailments and disease.

Sitting and Stilling the Mind: Taoist technique for calming and quieting the mind.

Six Healing Sounds: Six simple sounds, subvocalized during exhalation. Used to reduce heat in and heal the five major internal organs and the Triple Warmer.

Shen: The Third Treasure of Taoist Yoga. The mind. Also *Spirit.*

Slow Fire: Slow Abdominal Breathing.

Sperm Palace: A point on the male Functional Channel at the base of the penis under the pubic bone.

Spirit: The higher form of Shen. This is the part of us that Taoists believed could become Immortal.

Stove: The Lower Tan Tien. See *Warming the Stove.*

Superior Man (Woman): A person who cultivates his or her mind and moral character so as to act in harmony with the Tao.

Tai Chi: Unity. Also balance or harmony between two opposites.

Tan Tien: Literally "elixir" or "medicine" field. There are three in the body: Upper, Lower, and Middle. These are areas in which healing energies are produced or converted into other forms of energy, i.e. Jing into Chi or Chi into Shen.

Tao: The Way. The unknowable source of all that is, ever was or ever will be. Not really definable. Tao is a symbol rather than a name for that which is unnameable.

Tao In: Taoist calisthenics combining physical movement, stretching and breath. Taoist equivalent of Hatha Yoga.

Taoist Canon (Tao Tsang): More than two hundred thousand pages of the collected writings of Taoists from 500 B.C. to A.D. 1400. Only fragments have been translated into English.

Taoist Yoga: Taoist techniques for improving the health, rejuvenating the body, increasing longevity and making better use of sexuality.

Testicle Breathing: Male sexual practice for raising unaroused Sexual Energy to the brain.

Third Eye Point (Yin Tang): A point on the Governor Channel between and slightly above the two eyes.

Three Peaks of Great Medicine: Three parts of a woman's body believed to have healing and balancing qualities for her male partner. They are the tongue, the nipples and the vagina.

Three Pumps: Used to raise Jing or Chi up the spine and into the head. They are the perineum, the Sacral Pump and the Cranial Pump.

Three Treasures: The three basic components of Taoist Yoga: Chi, Jing and Shen (breath, body, and mind).

Third Treasure (Shen): Mind or Spirit. The third basic component of Taoist Yoga.

Tiger Cavity: A point in the palm of the left hand located by bending the middle finger into the palm. Used to absorb or send out Energy (Chi).

Tongue Kung Fu: Taoist sexual techniques using the tongue.

Triple Warmer: The three regions of the body, upper, middle, and lower. Considered an organ in Chinese Traditional Medicine, but is not an organ as understood in the West. Regulates body temperature.

Two Front Gates: Two "gates" in the sexual organs where Jing Chi (Sexual Energy) can be lost. In men they are at the tip and base of the penis. In women, the lips of the vagina and the urogenital diaphragm.

Upper Tan Tien: See *Crystal Palace.*

Vital Energy (Force): See *Original Chi (Yuan Chi).*

Warming the Stove: Raising the temperature of the Lower Tan Tien.

Water: One of the Five Elements (Five Forces). Cold energy. It is associated with the kidneys and sexual organs. Its color is black or sapphire blue.

Wei Dan: Physical exercises such as the Eight Pieces of Brocade, Tao In, calisthenics, weight-lifting, running, aerobics, etc.

Wei Kung: External Power. Strength gained from doing physical exercises such as the Eight Pieces of Brocade, Tao In, calisthenics, weight-lifting, running, aerobics, etc.

Wind: Air or gasses inside the body.

Wood: One of the Five Elements (Five Forces). Moist, warm energy. It is associated with the liver. Its color is emerald green.

Yang: The active aspect of any thought, idea, concept, energy, action, activity, etc. Often thought of as male, light, or positive.

Yi Chin Ching (The Muscle Tendon Change Classic): Chi Kung exercises designed to strengthen the muscles, soften and "grow" the tendons.

Yi Mind (Wisdom Mind): The higher mind. Ruled by the will, the intellect and intuition rather than the emotions. It is used to direct Chi within the body. Its seat is in the brain rather than the heart.

Yin: The passive or receptive aspect of any thought, idea, concept, energy, action, activity, etc. Often thought of as female, dark, or negative.

Yin Tang: See *Third Eye Point.*

bibliography

Burke, William R. *Chinese Healing Arts*. Burbank, CA: Unique Publications, 1986.

Chang, Stephen T. *The Great Tao*. Tao Publishing, 1985.

Chia, Mantak. *Awaken Healing Energy Through the Tao*. New York: Aurora Press, 1983.

Chia, Mantak and Michael Winn. *Taoist Secrets of Love Cultivating Male Sexual Energy*. New York: Aurora Press, 1984.

———. *Taoist Ways to Transform Stress Into Vitality*. New York: Healing Tao Press, 1985.

———. *Chi-Self Massage*. New York: Healing Tao Press, 1986.

Chia, Mantak and Maneewan Chia. *Healing Love Through the Tao: Cultivating Female Sexual Energy*. New York: Healing Tao Press, 1986.

———. *Iron Shirt Chi Kung*. New York: Healing Tao Press, 1986.

———. *Bone Marrow Nei Kung*. New York: Healing Tao Press, 1988.

———. *Fusion of the Five Elements I*. New York: Healing Tao Press, 1989.

———. *Chi Nei Tsang Internal Organs Massage*. New York: Healing Tao Press, 1990.

———. *Awaken Healing Light of the Tao*. New York: Healing Tao Press, 1993.

Chinese National Chi Kung Institute, eds. *Chi Kung Correspondence Program, Preliminary Instructions through Level Nine*. Moultan, AL: Chinese National Chi Kung Institute, 1986.

Cleary, Thomas. *The Secret of the Golden Flower*. San Francisco: Harper, 1991.

Chu, Valentin. *The Yin-Yang Butterfly*. New York: Tarcher/Putnam Book, 1993.

Deng Ming-Dao. *Scholar Warrior*. San Francisco: HarperCollins, 1990.

Guori, Jiao. *Qigong Essentials for Health Promotion*. Beijing, China: China Today Press, 1990.

Huang, Jane. *The Primordial Breath-Volume II*. Torrance,CA: Original Books, 1990.

Huang, Jane and Michael Wurmbrand. *The Primordial Breath-Volume I*. Torrance, CA: Original Books, 1987.

Jou, Tsung Hwa. *The Tao of Meditation*. Warwick, NY: Tai Chi Foundation, 1983.

Johnson, Jerry Alan. *The Essence of Internal Martial Arts–Volume II*. Pacific Grove, CA: Ching Lien Healing Arts Center, 1994.

Luk, Charles (Lu K'uan Yu). *The Secrets of Chinese Meditation*. New York: Samuel Weiser, 1964.

————. *Taoist Yoga*. New York: Samuel Weiser, 1970.

Ming, Dr. Yang Jwing. *The Root of Chinese Chi Kung*. Jamaica Plain, MA: Yang's Martial Arts Association, 1989.

————. *Muscle/Tendon Changing and Marrow/Brain Washing Chi Kung*. Jamaica Plain, MA: Yang's Martial Arts Association, 1989.

Zhang Mingwu and Sun Xingyuan. *Chinese Qigong Therapy*. Jinan, China: Shandong Science and Technology Press, 1985.

New World Press, eds. *Traditional Chinese Fitness Exercises*. Beijing, China: New World Press, 1984.

Hua-Ching Ni. *Attune Your Body with Dao-In*, Revised Edition. Santa Monica, CA: SevenStar Communications, 1994.

Reid, Daniel P. *The Tao of Health, Sex and Longevity*. New York: Fireside Book, 1989.

Chen Yan-feng. *Prenatal Energy Mobilising Qigong–China Taoist Ancient Qiqong*. Guangzou, China: Guangdong Science and Technology Press, 1992.

Yudelove, Eric Steven. *The Tao and the Tree of Life*. St. Paul, MN: Llewellyn Publications, 1995.

Walker, Brian. *Hua Hu Ching, The Unknown Teachings of Lao Tzu*. San Francisco, CA: Harper SanFrancisco, 1992.

Ware, James R. *Alchemy, Medicine and Religion in the China of A.D. 320, The Nei Pien of Ko Hung*. New York: Dover Publications, 1966.

Wile, Douglas. *The Art of the Bedchamber—The Chinese Sexual Yoga Classics Including Women's Solo Meditation Texts*. Albany, NY: State University of New York Press, 1992.

Wilhelm, Richard. *The Secret of the Golden Flower*. New York: Harvest Books, 1931.

———. *The I Ching or Book of Changes*. Princeton University Press, 1950.

Zong Wu and Li Mao. *Exercises Illustrated: Ancient Way to Keep Fit*. Hong Kong: Hai Feng Publishing Co., 1990.

H. F. Xue. *Pa Tuan Chin—Chinese Health Giving Exercise*. Hong Kong: Wan Li Book Co., 1988.

index

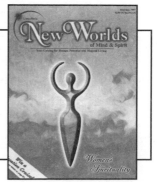

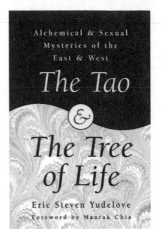

THE TAO & THE TREE OF LIFE
Alchemical & Sexual Mysteries of the East & West
Eric Steven Yudelove
Foreword by Mantak Chia

Until 1981, Taoist Yoga, or Taoist Internal Alchemy, remained a secret to the Western World. All of that changed when Master Mantak Chia emigrated from Thailand to the United States and began practicing openly. The complete Taoist Yoga system is now revealed—by one of Master Chia's first American students—in *The Tao and The Tree of Life*. Going beyond any previously published work, this book describes the entire structure of Taoist Yoga by comparing it with the Western Tradition of the Kaballah.

The Taoists developed the potential of human sexuality to a higher level than any other group. Uncover the secrets of single and dual cultivation, self-intercourse and the immortal child, as well as other mystical techniques never before available. Journey safely into the unknown through guided practice. Beginners can benefit almost immediately from the practical exercises in *The Tao and the Tree of Life*. Seasoned Kabbalists will marvel at actual alchemical formulas uncovered from The Sepher Yetzirah. There is a growing trend among Western Kabbalists to absorb the lower formulas of Taoist Yoga into their Tradition, and on the cusp of this rising tide is *The Tao and the Tree of Life*.

1-56718-250-X, 256 pp., 5 1/4 x 8, illus., softcover $14.95

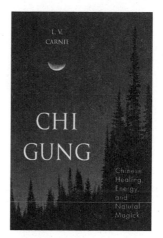

CHI GUNG
Chinese Healing, Energy and Natural Magick
L.V. Carnie

Chi Gung is unlike any other magickal book that you've read. There are no spells, incantations or special outfits. Instead, you will learn more than 80 different exercises that will help you to tap into the magickal power of universal energy. This power, called *Chi* in Chinese, permeates everything in existence; you can direct the flow of Chi to help you achieve ultimate health as well as any of your dreams and desires.

Chi Gung uses breathing, postures, and increased sensory awareness exercises that follow a particular training program. Ultimately, you can manipulate Chi without focusing on your breathing or moving your muscles in specific patterns. In fact, eventually you can learn how to move and transmit Chi instantly, anywhere, anytime, using only your mind. By learning the art of Chi Gung, you can slow the aging process; alter your metabolism; talk to plants and animals; move objects with your mind; withstand cold, heat and pain; and even read someone's soul.

1-56718-113-9, 7 x 10, 256 pp., illus., softcover $17.95

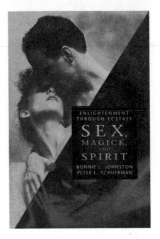

SEX, MAGICK, AND SPIRIT
Enlightenment Through Ecstasy
Bonnie L. Johnston and Peter L. Schuerman

Sex is a potent method for directing and releasing magical energies. The sexual act unites the polarities that exist within us, creating a strong current of energy which can be used to transform consciousness.

Sex, Magick, and Spirit is the first book to discuss the Sexual Mysteries of Western culture in a way that is relevant to modern times. It is for those who are interested in sacred sexuality but feel alienated by Eastern-based Tantra, and for Tantric practitioners who are interested in alternative approaches. You do not have to study Eastern philosophy or religious thought to practice the exercises described in this book.

Here you will learn the more advanced and esoteric aspects of sex. In going this next step, you leave behind the efforts to make sex safe and comfortable, and enter an exhilarating and sometimes disquieting realm in which sex is used to explore the very nature of your being.

1-56718-378-6, 7 x 10, 264 pp., illus. $17.95

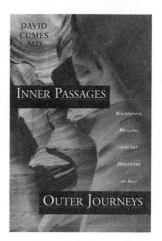

INNER PASSAGES
OUTER JOURNEYS
Wilderness, Healing and the Discovery of Self
David Cumes, M.D.

Whether you scale the sides of mountains or just putter in the garden, wilderness healer David Cumes, M.D., shows you how nature can be one of the most powerful and accessible forms of self-healing.

Few are prepared to commit to the rigors of disciplined spiritual practice. It is through nature that we can connect with our higher self most easily. The outer wilderness helps us access the inner wilderness of our psyches. When approached with the right frame of mind, wilderness can facilitate "peak experiences."

This book is for those with an adventurous spirit who may or may not have defined their spiritual path. It addresses the psychospiritual, healing and restorative effects of nature, and describes how to amplify your experience through transformational practices. This book is the first of its kind to combine the spirituality of the last surviving hunter gatherers of Africa with the ancient wisdom of yoga, Kabbala and shamanism.

1-56718-195-3, 6 x 9, 192 pp., illus. $12.95

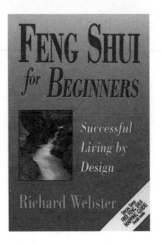

FENG SHUI FOR BEGINNERS
Successful Living by Design
Richard Webster

Not advancing fast enough in your career? Maybe your desk is located in a
"negative position." Wish you had a more peaceful family life? Hang a mirror in your dining room and watch what happens. Is money flowing out of
your life rather than into it? You may want to look to the construction of
your staircase!

For thousands of years, the ancient art of feng shui has helped people
harness universal forces and lead lives rich in good health, wealth and happiness. The basic techniques in *Feng Shui for Beginners* are very simple, and
you can put them into place immediately in your home and work environ-
ments. Gain peace of mind, a quiet confidence, and turn adversity to your
advantage with feng shui remedies.

1-56718-803-6, 240 pgs., 5 1/4 x 8, photos, diagrams, softcover $12.95